CHAIR YOGA FOR WEIGHT LOSS

A STEP-BY-STEP GUIDE TO MELT BELLY FAT AND ENHANCE YOUR WELLNESS WITH 10-MINUTE-A-DAY WORKOUTS | INCLUDES VIDEO TUTORIALS FOR EACH EXERCISE & 5 EXCLUSIVE BONUSES

LAURA SWITZER

TABLE OF CONTENTS

INTRODUCTION

Welcome to Chair Yoga for Weight Loss

Welcome to the world of Chair Yoga for Weight Loss, where the ancient wisdom of yoga meets the modern need for accessibility and ease. This practice is a gentle yet effective pathway to shedding unwanted pounds, gaining muscle tone, and enhancing overall wellness, all from the comfort of a chair. Whether you are a beginner just starting your fitness journey or someone who faces physical constraints that make traditional yoga challenging, chair yoga offers a welcoming and inclusive alternative.

Chair yoga, by its design, is a perfect fit for individuals of all ages and fitness levels. It strips away the barriers of intensive physical workouts and introduces a method that is accessible to everyone—regardless of physical condition or age. In this approach, the chair is not just a prop but a supportive partner in your journey towards health and weight loss. It helps maintain balance, provides stability, and allows you to perform yoga poses with greater confidence and less risk of injury.

Chair yoga's beauty is in how simple it is and how profoundly it can work on the body. It works on specific muscle groups that are important for metabolism and fat burning through a series of seated and standing poses. With regular practice, it can aid with weight reduction and gradually increase mobility and flexibility. The gentle movements involved in chair yoga also stimulate the digestive system, enhance blood circulation, and boost metabolic rates, all of which contribute to more effective weight management.

Moreover, chair yoga is not just about physical benefits; it also encompasses mental and emotional gains. Each session is an opportunity to reduce stress and foster a sense of inner peace, both of which are vital in the modern, fast-paced world. Stress reduction is particularly important in managing belly fat—a common trouble area for many. The cortisol hormone, which is released in response to stress, is linked to increased abdominal fat. Through mindful breathing and relaxation techniques incorporated into chair yoga, you can manage stress better and, consequently, reduce belly fat.

Embracing chair yoga means setting up a small, dedicated space that invites calm and concentration. This doesn't require a large studio or an array of expensive equipment; a quiet corner of your home with just enough space for a chair and free movement is sufficient. The key is to create an environment that motivates you to practice regularly. Equally important is choosing the right chair. Ensure that it is sturdy without arms, allowing freedom of movement for various poses. The right equipment can transform your practice, making each pose more effective and enjoyable.

Each session of chair yoga brings a promise of renewal and revitalization. As you stretch and move, even in a limited space, you begin to break down the mental barriers that associate fitness and wellbeing with vigorous, floor-based exercises. Chair yoga teaches you to find opportunities for health and vitality in stillness and small movements, redefining what effective exercise looks like for you.

The goal of chair yoga is to help you understand your body and its requirements better than merely helping you lose weight. It's about creating harmony between your physical actions and mental intentions, where every gentle stretch and each deep breath aligns you closer to your wellness goals. As you continue with this practice, you'll notice not just a transformation in your body but also an enhanced capacity for joy and a renewed vigor for life.

As we embark on this journey together in this guide, remember that every movement is a step forward in your path to health. With each pose, you'll discover not only the strength and flexibility of your body but also the resilience and adaptability of your spirit. Chair yoga is not just an exercise routine; it's a celebration of what your body can do, no matter your starting point. As you progress, this form of yoga will continue to be a source of support and strength, helping you achieve a healthier, lighter you in a way that respects your body's limits and expands its horizons.

How to Use This Book

This book is designed to be a comprehensive guide for anyone looking to integrate chair yoga into their daily routine to aid weight loss and improve overall health. As you navigate through the pages, you will find a structured approach to practicing yoga with the aid of a chair, making the exercises accessible and effective for individuals of all ages and fitness levels. To enhance your experience and ensure you get the most out of every session, this guide includes several features, such as QR codes and video tutorials, that will assist you in understanding and performing the exercises correctly.

To begin, it's important to familiarize yourself with the layout of the book. Each chapter is carefully crafted to gradually introduce you to the concepts and exercises of chair yoga, starting with the basics and moving towards more advanced techniques. This progression is designed to help you build strength and flexibility at a comfortable pace, ensuring that each new exercise adds to your ability without overwhelming you.

The inclusion of QR codes throughout the book is a key feature designed to enrich your learning experience. These codes can be easily scanned with a smartphone or a tablet, directing you to online video tutorials related to the exercises being discussed. Watching a video demonstration can clarify the textual descriptions, giving you a better understanding of the posture and movement techniques, which are crucial for preventing injuries and maximizing the benefits of the exercises.

Integrating these video tutorials into your practice is straightforward. As you read through the descriptions of each exercise, take a moment to scan the accompanying QR code and watch the video. This will help you visualize the movements and the proper alignments before you try them out yourself. It's recommended that you watch the videos in a quiet space where you can focus and possibly follow along in real time. This dual approach of reading and watching will cater to different learning preferences and reinforce your understanding of how each pose should be executed.

In addition to learning the exercises, this book encourages you to incorporate chair yoga into your daily routine. This doesn't mean you need to carve out large segments of your day; instead, it's about finding small windows of opportunity to practice. Even ten minutes a day can be beneficial, especially when done consistently. Consider starting or ending your day with a few stretches and poses, or use them as a productive break from sitting at your desk. Regular practice is key to achieving the health benefits and weight loss goals associated with chair yoga.

Furthermore, the video tutorials offer more than just exercise demonstrations. They often include modifications to adapt each pose to different fitness levels and physical conditions. This ensures that you can participate safely and effectively, regardless of your current ability or mobility. Pay attention to these modifications and apply them as needed to tailor the workouts to your personal needs.

As you progress through the book, try to keep a journal of your experiences. Note any changes in how you feel physically and mentally, as well as any particular poses that you find beneficial or challenging. This record can serve as a motivational tool and help you track your progress over time. It can also guide you in adjusting your practice to better suit your evolving fitness levels and health goals.

Lastly, remember that consistency is crucial. Make chair yoga a part of your routine, and you will likely see improvements not just in your physical health but also in your overall wellbeing. Use this book as a daily companion, refer back to the video tutorials whenever you need a refresher, and continue to explore the deeper aspects of yoga as you advance through the chapters.

With the help of the tools and resources included in this book, which include video lessons, QR codes, and written descriptions, you will be well-prepared to start your path toward a transforming practice with chair yoga. Whether your objective is to become more flexible, shed some pounds, or just find a new method to unwind and reduce stress, this book will help you every step of the way to make your practice successful and pleasurable.

CHAPTER 1

A DEEP DIVE INTO CHAIR YOGA

Understanding Chair Yoga

A modified version of yoga known as chair yoga enables practitioners to do poses while seated or with the assistance of a chair. With this technique, yoga becomes accessible to anyone who might otherwise find it difficult because of age-related concerns, mobility problems, or physical restrictions. Yoga practitioners can benefit from improved flexibility, improved balance, and increased strength by using a chair instead of standing or doing a lot of floor work to achieve traditional poses.

The primary components of chair yoga revolve around modifications of standard yoga poses. These adaptations make the practices suitable for sitting or using the chair for support during standing poses. For instance, a traditional pose like the Warrior can be performed with the aid of a chair to maintain balance, ensuring that even those who cannot stand for long periods can still engage in strengthening their muscles and improving their posture.

A variety of motions and exercises created especially to extend the range of motion are included in chair yoga. These movements target various parts of the body, from the neck and shoulders to the legs and feet. Because the exercises can be adjusted to individual needs and abilities, chair yoga is exceptionally versatile, catering to people at different fitness levels and with various health conditions.

One of the significant advantages of chair yoga is its effectiveness in promoting weight loss. While it might seem less intense than other forms of exercise, chair yoga can help raise the heart rate and boost metabolism, both of which are crucial for burning calories. Repeated motions in the sequences serve to improve the efficiency of fat burning by increasing oxygen and blood supply to the muscles. The body burns more calories at rest thanks to the muscle-building benefits of these positions, which also raise basal metabolic rate.

In addition to aiding in weight loss, chair yoga improves overall health in several ways. Firstly, it enhances flexibility. Frequent muscular stretching can improve the range of motion, lessen stiffness, and lessen discomfort from ailments like back issues or arthritis. The gentle nature of chair yoga makes these stretches easy to perform without the risk of injury that might come with more vigorous exercise.

Furthermore, chair yoga is known for its ability to reduce stress and promote mental clarity. Each session typically incorporates breathing exercises, which can help calm the mind and reduce anxiety. Along with its own advantages, mental relaxation also improves blood pressure, sleep quality, and immunological function, all of which are important for general physical health.

The practice also emphasizes balance and proprioception, which is the awareness of the body's position in space. Improving balance is particularly important for older adults as it can help prevent falls. By strengthening the core and improving coordination, chair yoga helps individuals maintain their independence and mobility as they age.

For those looking to integrate chair yoga into their daily routine, the flexibility of the practice makes it easy to adapt. It can be practiced in various settings, from the office to the living room, making it a convenient option for those with busy schedules or limited access to traditional yoga studios. Each session can be as short or as long as desired, with even a few minutes of practice providing beneficial effects.

Additionally, chair yoga promotes a holistic approach to health. It encourages practitioners to consider their physical, mental, and emotional wellbeing as interconnected aspects of their overall health. This holistic perspective can lead to more sustained health improvements as individuals learn to listen to their bodies and address needs that go beyond simple physical fitness.

The Origins and Evolution of Chair Yoga

Chair yoga, while a relatively modern adaptation in the Western world, is rooted in the ancient practices of yoga that originated over 5,000 years ago in India. Yoga itself has always been an evolving practice designed to meet the spiritual, mental, and physical needs of its practitioners. As yoga traveled across continents and cultures, it transformed and adapted, leading to the development of various styles and forms, including chair yoga, which addresses the needs of those who might find traditional yoga poses challenging.

The origins of chair yoga can be traced back to the necessity for making yoga accessible to all, regardless of physical limitations or age. While there is no specific point in history where chair yoga was officially created, it is a natural evolution of the practice's foundational goal: to make the physical and mental benefits of yoga universally accessible. This adaptation is particularly significant as it aligns with yoga's core principles of inclusivity and adaptability.

In the late 20th century, as yoga began to gain popularity in the West, there was a growing awareness of its potential health benefits, not just as a form of exercise but as a holistic tool for wellness and therapeutic purposes. This period saw yoga teachers and therapists exploring ways to modify traditional poses to accommodate those who could not participate in standard yoga classes. These individuals included the elderly, those with disabilities, and others with conditions that limited their mobility. It was from this need that chair yoga began to take shape, using a chair as a tool to perform yoga poses safely and effectively.

The chair serves multiple purposes in this form of yoga. It acts as an extension of the body, offering support and stability, which allows practitioners to perform stretches and poses with more control and less strain. The chair also enables practitioners to focus on their breath and alignment without worrying about balance, making the practice more accessible and less intimidating for beginners or those with physical challenges.

As chair yoga continued to evolve, it was incorporated into various therapeutic settings, including hospitals, senior centers, and rehabilitation clinics. Medical professionals and yoga therapists recognize its benefits in improving flexibility, strength, and mental clarity, which are crucial for the elderly and those recovering from injuries or dealing with chronic pain. This acknowledgment further propelled the popularity and acceptance of chair yoga within the health and wellness community.

Today, chair yoga is celebrated for its versatility and inclusivity. It has been adapted for office settings, where individuals can perform brief sessions to alleviate the physical and mental strains of prolonged sitting. Schools use chair yoga to help students manage stress and increase their concentration. Moreover, chair yoga classes are now a regular feature in many traditional yoga studios, offering an alternative for those who wish to practice yoga in a more supportive setting.

The modern adaptations of chair yoga also reflect a broader shift towards personalized wellness, where fitness and health practices are tailored to meet individual needs and lifestyles. This shift acknowledges that health and wellness are not one-size-fits-all and that practices like yoga need to be adaptable to be truly beneficial.

The evolution of chair yoga is a testament to the adaptability and resilience of the practice of yoga itself. It embodies the principle that yoga is not merely a physical exercise but a lifestyle that enhances wellbeing at all levels. Chair yoga has opened the door for many who would otherwise find it difficult to engage in traditional yoga, providing a pathway to improved health and increased vitality.

Chair yoga's journey from a niche modification to a mainstream practice underscores a broader cultural recognition of the importance of accessibility in health and wellness. It continues to evolve, driven by innovative teachers and therapists who are exploring new ways to make yoga even more inclusive. As chair yoga moves forward, it carries with it the essence of yoga's ancient wisdom, proving that the core principles of yoga can be adapted to meet the changing needs of society. Its continued evolution and growing popularity highlight an ongoing commitment to ensuring that the profound benefits of yoga are available to everyone, no matter their circumstances.

How Chair Yoga Differs from Traditional Yoga Practices

Chair yoga is a significant modification of traditional yoga that benefits and is accessible to a wider range of people, including those with special needs or restricted mobility. Traditional yoga, known for its various poses and practices aimed at enhancing physical, mental, and spiritual health, often requires a level of flexibility, balance, and strength that may not be feasible for everyone. Chair yoga, by contrast, modifies these poses to make them achievable for people who may find floor exercises challenging.

The essence of traditional yoga involves a series of poses (asanas), breath control (pranayama), and meditation (dhyana), all aimed at harmonizing the body and mind. These practices are typically performed on a yoga mat, with various levels of complexity and intensity, depending on the style of yoga. However, for individuals dealing with conditions like arthritis, osteoporosis, or balance issues, or for those who are elderly, these traditional poses can be difficult and sometimes risky.

By modifying these classic poses to be performed while seated in a chair or utilizing the chair as a support, chair yoga provides a kind substitute. This method makes yoga practice safer and more accessible by reducing joint and muscle strain in addition to supplying stability and balance. To decrease the amount of balance and strength needed, one can modify a conventional posture like the Warrior by doing it while seated or by utilizing the chair to support a portion of the body's weight.

One of the primary differences between chair yoga and traditional yoga is the level of physical exertion required. Traditional yoga often involves transitions between standing, seated, and lying positions, which can be strenuous for some. Chair yoga minimizes these movements, focusing instead on upper body movements, gentle stretching, and deep breathing, all done within the safety and comfort of a chair. This makes it ideal not only for those with physical limitations but also for people recovering from surgery or illness, providing them with a means to maintain mobility and flexibility without undue stress on their bodies.

Another key difference lies in the accessibility of chair yoga. Traditional yoga classes may sometimes seem intimidating to beginners or those unsure about their physical capabilities, particularly in classes where more advanced poses are practiced. Chair yoga classes, on the other hand, often foster a more inclusive atmosphere, where the focus is on what each individual can do rather than on what they cannot. This inclusivity encourages a diverse range of participants, each able to modify the practice to suit their comfort and ability levels.

Additionally, chair yoga can be particularly beneficial for those who spend long hours seated, such as office workers or drivers, who may suffer from poor posture and its associated pains. Traditional yoga does offer poses that can help with these issues, but not everyone may feel comfortable performing all traditional poses. Chair yoga provides these individuals with practical exercises that can be performed even in an office setting, helping to alleviate back pain, improve posture, and enhance concentration.

Moreover, chair yoga emphasizes the meditative and breath control aspects of yoga, which are integral to traditional practices. By focusing on deep, mindful breathing, chair yoga helps reduce stress and anxiety, enhance lung capacity, and improve overall vitality. These benefits are accessible without the need for complex poses or extensive physical strength, making the mental health benefits of yoga available to a broader audience.

The Science of Weight Loss with Chair Yoga

Chair yoga, often perceived as a gentle and accessible form of yoga, holds significant potential for aiding weight loss, particularly for those who find traditional exercise challenging due to age, mobility, or health issues. This form of yoga not only provides a low-impact way to engage in physical activity but also stimulates metabolism, thereby contributing effectively to weight loss.

Comprehending the function of metabolism in the body's energy regulation is the first step toward comprehending how chair yoga contributes to weight loss. All of the biochemical reactions that take place in our bodies, including the ones that convert food's nutrients into energy, are referred to as metabolism. An active metabolism efficiently burns calories, not only during physical activity but also at rest. Chair yoga helps boost metabolism by combining physical postures with controlled breathing, which together enhance the efficiency of both the respiratory and cardiovascular systems.

Engaging in chair yoga involves a series of movements and stretches that increase muscle activity. Even though these activities are performed while seated or using a chair for support, they require muscle engagement similar to that in mild to moderate exercise. For example, performing a seated version of the Warrior pose involves extending the arms and holding the position, which activates the muscles in the arms, shoulders, and back. Such sustained muscle activity increases energy expenditure, which, over time, contributes to weight loss.

Chair yoga also enhances muscular tone. Muscles need energy even when you are not moving since they are metabolically active tissues. Chair yoga increases your basal metabolic rate (BMR), or the rate at which your body burns calories when at rest, by toning your muscles. Even when you are not actively exercising, having a higher basal metabolic rate (BMR) might help you lose weight since it indicates that your body utilizes more energy throughout the day.

Breathing exercises, or pranayama, which are a core component of chair yoga, also play a crucial role in enhancing metabolic function. Deep, mindful breathing increases oxygen intake and improves blood circulation. Better oxygenation of blood ensures that more oxygen reaches the muscles and organs, enhancing their function and boosting metabolism. Pranayama also helps in stress reduction, which is crucial because stress can lead to hormonal imbalances that might increase weight gain through mechanisms like increased appetite and fat storage, particularly abdominal fat.

Furthermore, chair yoga promotes better digestion, another key factor in weight management. Many chair yoga poses involve gentle twisting and bending movements that massage the abdominal organs. By stimulating the digestive system, these motions can aid in better nutritional absorption and digestion as well as aid in the body's removal of waste and pollutants. An efficient digestive system reduces bloating and helps maintain a healthy weight.

Chair yoga also impacts weight loss through its effects on insulin sensitivity. Yoga has been demonstrated to increase insulin sensitivity on a regular basis, which helps the body better control blood sugar levels. Improved insulin sensitivity not only helps in preventing and managing diabetes but also discourages the body from storing excess glucose as fat, thus aiding in weight loss.

Chair yoga's psychological advantages, such as improved concentration and reduced anxiety, can support weight loss. Anxiety and stress can cause emotional eating and make bad nutritional decisions. Chair yoga techniques build mindfulness, which can improve weight reduction attempts by managing stress and lowering the chance of stress-related eating.

Metabolic Benefits: How Gentle Movements Can Lead to Weight Loss

Engaging in chair yoga, characterized by its gentle movements and accessibility, initiates a series of physiological changes within the body that contribute significantly to weight loss and enhanced metabolism. This seemingly modest form of exercise is powerful in its ability to transform health, particularly for those who may be restricted by physical conditions that make more vigorous forms of exercise challenging.

Chair yoga primarily affects the body through increased metabolic rate, enhanced muscle efficiency, and improved endocrine function. These physiological changes are crucial for weight loss and overall health enhancement. When practicing chair yoga, even the gentlest movements require muscle engagement. These movements, though mild, are significant enough to stimulate muscle fibers, particularly in the core, arms, and legs. As muscles engage, they consume energy. The more muscle tissue involved in an activity, the more calories are burned, not only during the exercise but also at rest, because muscle tissue is metabolically active.

The increased muscle activity during chair yoga poses leads to enhanced circulation. As muscles contract and relax, they push blood back towards the heart, improving overall circulation. Better circulation increases the amount of oxygen and nutrients that reach all of the body's tissues, improving metabolism and cell function. Better-oxygenated cells operate more effectively, which raises the metabolic rate. Oxygen is necessary for the metabolic processes that turn food into energy.

Another significant physiological change induced by chair yoga involves the enhancement of endocrine function, particularly the balance of stress hormones such as cortisol. A key player in metabolism and the body's reaction to stress, cortisol is sometimes referred to as the stress hormone. Weight gain, particularly around the middle, and a sluggish metabolism might result from high cortisol levels. Stress and cortisol levels can be lowered by combining chair yoga's meditative elements with deliberate, deep breathing. By lowering cortisol, belly obesity can be avoided, and a more balanced metabolism can result.

Chair yoga also positively affects insulin sensitivity. Regular practice of these gentle movements can improve the body's response to insulin, the hormone responsible for regulating blood sugar levels. Improved insulin sensitivity means that the body is better able to use glucose from the bloodstream for energy rather than storing it as fat. This is particularly important for weight management and overall metabolic health, as high blood sugar levels can lead to fat storage and increase the risk of diabetes.

Furthermore, the practice of chair yoga stimulates the digestive system. Movements such as twisting and bending gently massage the internal organs, including the digestive tract. This massage improves the efficiency of the digestive system, helping to increase the rate at which the body processes and eliminates waste. A healthy, efficient digestive system is crucial for weight loss, as it helps to prevent bloating and constipation and ensures that nutrients are effectively absorbed and used by the body.

The mild motions of chair yoga are also beneficial to the lymphatic system, which is essential for both waste elimination and immunological function. The lymphatic system uses only bodily motions to circulate lymph fluid throughout the body, in contrast to the circulatory system, which uses the heart to pump blood. The stretching and compressing actions inherent in chair yoga poses help push lymph fluid through the body, enhancing the removal of toxins and boosting immune function. A well-functioning lymphatic system contributes to better health and supports metabolic processes.

The Role of Stress Reduction in Fighting Belly Fat

The battle against belly fat often extends beyond diet and exercise to include managing one's stress levels. Research consistently highlights stress as a significant factor in weight gain, particularly around the midsection. Yoga, especially practices like chair yoga that focus on deep breathing and relaxation, offers a powerful tool for stress reduction, which can directly influence the reduction of belly fat.

Stress sets off the body's fight-or-flight reaction, which releases cortisol, a hormone that is necessary for life but may be harmful if it is raised over an extended period of time. Because cortisol affects metabolism and fat storage, high levels have been associated with increased belly fat. Cortisol can promote the accumulation of unutilized resources, such as belly fat, and increase desire and cravings for meals rich in calories. This process was beneficial in evolutionary terms, providing energy reserves during times of stress, such as famine or flight situations, but in the context of modern chronic stress, it contributes to unwanted belly fat.

Chair yoga, with its gentle sequences and focus on mindful breathing, directly addresses stress. The practice of deep, controlled breathing is central to all forms of yoga and is particularly effective in activating the parasympathetic nervous system, the body's natural relaxation response.

This is in contrast to the sympathetic nervous system, which releases cortisol when under stress. By engaging the parasympathetic nervous system, chair yoga helps lower cortisol levels, thereby reducing the physiological impulse to accumulate belly fat.

Furthermore, the mindfulness cultivated through yoga practice can alter one's emotional relationship with food and eating habits, which are often disrupted by stress. Regular yoga practice fosters a greater awareness of bodily sensations and emotional states, which can help individuals recognize stress-induced cravings for what they are rather than genuine hunger signals. This awareness can reduce instances of emotional eating, a common response to stress that typically involves high-calorie, unhealthy foods that contribute to belly fat.

The physical postures in chair yoga also play a role in combating belly fat. Although the movements are gentle, they involve core strengthening and elongation, which improve posture and muscle tone in the abdominal area. A stronger core can indirectly aid in the appearance and reduction of belly fat by improving overall body alignment and the efficiency of movements during daily activities, leading to increased calorie burn.

Chair yoga's sequences also improve overall digestion and help to stimulate the metabolism, both of which are adversely affected by stress. Stress can slow down the digestive process, leading to bloating and discomfort, which exacerbates the appearance of belly fat. The twisting and bending movements common in yoga massage internal organs, including the digestive tract, enhance blood flow, help to process food more efficiently, and eliminate toxins, which are factors important in managing weight and reducing belly fat.

In addition to physiological benefits, the mental and emotional relief provided by chair yoga encourages a healthier lifestyle overall. Regular practitioners often report better sleep patterns, more energy, and a more positive outlook—factors that contribute to a healthier lifestyle and better choices. Better sleep, in particular, is associated with reduced levels of ghrelin, the hunger hormone, and increased levels of leptin, the hormone responsible for signaling fullness. Adequate sleep, therefore, helps regulate appetite and can reduce cravings that lead to belly fat.

Chair yoga's holistic approach to stress reduction, involving both mind and body, makes it an effective practice for those struggling with belly fat. By reducing cortisol levels, enhancing mindfulness, improving digestion and metabolism, strengthening the core, and promoting better sleep and healthier lifestyle choices, chair yoga addresses many of the direct and indirect causes of belly fat. This makes it more than just an exercise; it is a comprehensive strategy for improving health and reducing one of the most stubborn and harmful types of body fat.

Creating a Conducive Environment

Creating a conducive environment for yoga at home is vital to enhance the practice's benefits and make it a calming and supportive experience. The right setting can significantly influence your ability to relax, focus, and fully engage with the yoga poses and breathing exercises.

Start by choosing a quiet corner of your home where interruptions are minimal. This space should be away from high-traffic areas to ensure peace and tranquility. Adequate space is essential, so make sure there is enough room to move freely in all directions. The physical boundaries of your yoga area are as crucial as its ambiance. It doesn't need to be large; just ensure it's sufficient to stretch out fully, both vertically and horizontally.

Next, consider the lighting. Natural light is ideal, promoting a sense of freshness and vitality. If possible, set up near a window that offers soft, natural sunlight. However, if you practice yoga in the evening, ensure the lighting is soothing and not too harsh or glaring. Soft, warm artificial lights can create a serene atmosphere that enhances your practice.

The surface you practice on is also important. A yoga mat is ideal because it cushions your body and provides grip for your feet and hands. Choose a mat that feels comfortable and supports your joints, especially if you're doing seated or reclining poses that require you to be on the floor for extended periods.

Personalize your space to make it more inviting and relaxing. This could include adding elements such as a small indoor plant, calming artwork, or a simple statue that inspires peace or mindfulness. Background music can also be beneficial. Consider playing gentle, soothing tunes or nature sounds that help drown out distracting noise and set a meditative mood.

Preparing Your Space: Setting Up a Home Yoga Studio

Setting up a home yoga studio is an enriching project that can transform a part of your living space into a sanctuary for health and wellbeing. To start, identify a quiet area within your home where disturbances are minimal. This could be a spare room, a section of your bedroom, or a peaceful corner in a less frequented part of the house. Selecting a place where you can be private and won't be disturbed is crucial.

Once you have selected the space, consider the flooring. Hardwood floors are ideal for stability when performing poses, but if that's not available, any flat surface will do. Lay down a high-quality yoga mat that provides ample cushioning and grip to support your body and prevent slipping. If you anticipate doing more restorative sessions, having additional yoga props like blocks, bolsters, and a blanket can enhance your comfort and the effectiveness of your poses.

A home studio's ambiance is greatly influenced by its lighting. To keep the area light and airy during the day, try to let as much natural light as you can into the room. Install warm, soft lighting for nighttime rehearsals to assist in creating a relaxing atmosphere. Stay away from fluorescent lighting, as it can be glaring and distracting.

Air quality is also important. Ensure good ventilation to keep the room fresh, and consider adding plants that can purify the air naturally. A well-ventilated space helps maintain energy levels and deep breathing, which are crucial for effective yoga practice.

Personal touches will make the space inviting and inspire regular practice. Decorate with items that evoke serenity and peace, such as candles for soft lighting, inspirational quotes, or a small statue. Consider also incorporating elements of nature, like a bowl of shells or a small fountain, to bring tranquility to the environment.

Finally, keep the space clean and clutter-free. Regularly tidy up the area to preserve its calmness and readiness for practice. A dedicated and well-maintained space not only invites regular practice but also deepens your yoga experience, making every session at home a retreat into mindfulness and personal growth.

Choosing the Right Equipment: Chairs and Accessories for Effective Practice

Choosing the right equipment is crucial for enhancing your chair yoga practice, ensuring it is both effective and enjoyable. The central piece of equipment in chair yoga is, of course, the chair itself. Select a chair that is sturdy and stable without arms, allowing freedom of movement for various poses. The chair should have a flat seat that supports your entire sitting bones and a straight back to promote proper posture. Avoid chairs that are too soft or that recline, as they can make maintaining the correct posture difficult.

In addition to a suitable chair, consider investing in a few more accessories to enrich your practice. A yoga mat is essential, even for chair yoga, as it provides a grippy surface for your feet, ensuring stability during standing or seated poses that require you to place your feet on the ground. Opt for a mat with good cushioning to protect your joints, particularly if you perform any poses standing beside the chair.

Yoga blocks are another valuable accessory. They can be used to support your hands in poses where you can't quite reach the ground, helping to maintain alignment and balance. Yoga straps are useful for extending your reach and improving your flexibility, allowing you to hold onto your feet or legs in stretches without straining.

For those looking to deepen their relaxation during meditation and restorative poses, a yoga blanket can be a great addition. Fold it up to use as a cushion or to offer extra support under your knees or back. The blanket can also provide warmth during the final relaxation pose, helping you to fully relax and let go.

Lastly, consider the space around your chair. Ensure there is enough room to move freely without obstruction and keep your yoga accessories within easy reach. Creating an inviting and functional practice area will motivate you to use it regularly, enhancing both your physical flexibility and your mental wellbeing.

Dear Readers,

Thank you for starting this journey with us through the enriching practice of chair yoga. We hope that the techniques and insights presented in this first chapter have inspired you to embrace yoga as a part of your daily routine. If you found the information helpful, we would greatly appreciate it if you took a few moments to share your thoughts by leaving a review on Amazon. Your feedback is invaluable to us and helps others discover the benefits of this practice.

How You Can Share Your Review

Through Amazon.com:

1. Go to the Amazon page where you found my book.
2. Navigate to the 'Customer Reviews' section.
3. Click on 'Write a customer review' to share your valuable insights.

Instant QR Code Access: Simply scan the QR code below with your smartphone to be directed to the Amazon review section.

CHAPTER 2

THE HOLISTIC BENEFITS OF CHAIR YOGA

Beyond Weight Loss: How Chair Yoga Enhances Overall Wellbeing

Chair yoga is often celebrated for its accessibility and ease, making it an ideal exercise for those with physical limitations or those who spend much of their day seated. However, the benefits of chair yoga extend far beyond the mere physical, touching on aspects of mental and emotional health that are crucial for a balanced and healthy lifestyle.

One of the most significant benefits of chair yoga is its ability to reduce stress and anxiety. This is achieved through a combination of mindful breathing, gentle stretching, and the meditative focus that is central to all yoga practices. Chair yoga encourages participants to concentrate on their breath—a technique that helps calm the mind and ease the body's stress response. This type of deep, regular breathing balances the fight-or-flight response by stimulating the parasympathetic nerve system, which is in charge of the body's rest and digestive processes. By engaging this system, chair yoga helps to reduce overall stress levels, leading to improvements in mood and a decrease in anxiety symptoms.

Additionally, the slow, controlled movements required in chair yoga increase body awareness. This heightened awareness, also known as proprioception, helps participants become more attuned to their physical condition, posture, and alignment.

This awareness naturally extends beyond the yoga session itself, encouraging better posture and movement in daily activities, which can help alleviate common issues like back pain and muscle strain. This has the potential to significantly increase physical comfort and mobility over time, which are directly related to increases in mental health.

Chair yoga also promotes better sleep, a critical component of mental health. The relaxation and stress relief provided by regular yoga practice has been shown to help individuals fall asleep faster, sleep more deeply, and feel more rested upon waking. Since mood management, cognitive function, and overall health all depend on getting enough sleep, any exercise that helps with sleep is extremely helpful.

The practice of chair yoga can also enhance cognitive functions. The concentration required to perform and hold the poses, combined with the need to coordinate breathing and movement, can boost mental alertness and focus. Regular practice has been associated with improvements in memory, attention, and even executive functions like problem-solving and decision-making. For older adults, in particular, this can mean not only a better quality of life but also a delay in cognitive decline associated with aging.

Chair yoga helps people develop a stronger emotional bond with themselves. As a result, people may experience an increase in self-worth and acceptance as they come to recognize and value their bodies and skills in spite of any restrictions. Additionally, the practice frequently incorporates mindfulness and gratitude, which can help individuals focus on the good parts of their lives and change their perspective, ultimately increasing their level of life satisfaction.

Chair yoga also fosters a sense of community, even if practiced alone at home. Chair yoga practitioners frequently take online courses or join communities where they may exchange stories and encourage one another's development. This sense of belonging and community can be particularly powerful for those who might otherwise feel isolated due to physical limitations or age, adding a social component that greatly enhances emotional health.

Moreover, the adaptability of chair yoga means that it can continually be adjusted to meet the evolving needs of its practitioners. This adaptability not only helps in maintaining physical health regardless of age or ability level but also empowers individuals by giving them control over their wellness routine. This sense of empowerment is critical for mental health, contributing to a feeling of independence and self-efficacy.

Integration of Mind and Body: Mental Clarity

Chair yoga is much more than just a physical practice; it's a profound method for fostering an integration of mind and body that leads to enhanced mental clarity and focus. This form of yoga makes the meditative benefits of traditional yoga accessible to all, including those who may not be able to engage in more physically demanding forms. Through a series of gentle movements and focused breathing, chair yoga participants experience a mindfulness practice that brings significant mental benefits.

The mindfulness aspect of chair yoga starts with the breath. Breathing exercises, or pranayama, are central to the practice and help to quiet the mind and focus attention. These exercises encourage participants to breathe deeply and consciously, which increases oxygen flow to the brain, helping to clear mental fog and reduce cognitive stress. The act of focusing on the breath also helps center the mind, pulling attention away from distracting thoughts and anchoring it in the present moment. This enhanced focus is crucial not only during the yoga session but also in daily life as it improves the ability to concentrate on tasks and remain present in interactions.

Moreover, the specific poses and stretches in chair yoga require a level of attention and precision that further cultivates mindfulness. Each movement is performed deliberately and in sync with the breath, which reinforces the connection between physical actions and mental awareness. This practice of mindful movement teaches the brain to focus on what the body is experiencing from moment to moment, which can lead to improved mental clarity.

Participants often report that this heightened awareness continues beyond their yoga practice, helping them to maintain focus and clarity in their everyday activities.

Chair yoga also involves an element of meditation, which directly impacts mental clarity. Meditation practices embedded within the yoga session, such as guided imagery or silent reflection, encourage deep relaxation and mental stillness. These practices allow the mind to take a break from the constant stimulation of daily life, which is often filled with multitasking and digital interruptions. By providing a space for the mind to rest, chair yoga helps to reduce mental clutter and fatigue, leading to a refreshed and clear mental state.

The relaxation techniques practiced in chair yoga also play a significant role in achieving mental clarity. Stress is a common cause of mental confusion and scattered thoughts. The relaxation phase of chair yoga, typically at the end of a session, helps to significantly lower stress levels through deep relaxation of the body and mind. This not only alleviates stress but also enhances overall mental functioning, allowing for clearer thinking and better problem-solving abilities.

Furthermore, the holistic approach of chair yoga, which emphasizes physical health as a component of mental wellbeing, contributes to mental clarity. By improving physical health and alleviating physical discomforts such as pain or stiffness, chair yoga helps remove physical distractions that can cloud the mind. This connection between physical wellness and mental clarity is fundamental, as discomfort can significantly disrupt concentration and mental performance.

Regular practice of chair yoga builds resilience against the impacts of stress and anxiety, which are common culprits behind a muddled mind. The techniques learned and practiced in chair yoga sessions—such as mindful breathing, focused attention, and meditation—equip participants with tools they can use outside of yoga to manage stress and maintain mental clarity amidst life's challenges.

The community aspect of chair yoga should not be overlooked either in its contribution to mental clarity. Participating in chair yoga classes, even virtually, can create a sense of community and shared experience that enhances emotional wellbeing. Emotional health, strongly tied to mental clarity, benefits significantly from feelings of connection and belonging, which can reduce feelings of isolation or emotional distress that might cloud mental clarity.

Nutrition and Holistic Health

In order to maintain the physical practice of yoga and create a comprehensive approach to wellness that nourishes the body and mind, nutrition is essential. When paired with the mindful and restorative practice of yoga, a thoughtful and balanced diet can amplify the benefits of the exercises, improving not only physical strength and flexibility but also contributing to mental clarity and emotional balance.

Focusing on a diet that supplies the body with the necessary nutrients and meets the restorative and energetic demands of yoga is crucial to enhancing the physical components of the practice. This entails including a range of foods that offer a well-balanced combination of fats, proteins, and carbs in addition to vital vitamins and minerals to promote general health.

Carbohydrates are vital for energy, which is necessary to maintain the stamina required for yoga practices. However, choosing the right types of carbohydrates is key. Whole grains such as brown rice, quinoa, and oats are excellent sources of complex carbohydrates that release energy gradually, as opposed to simple carbohydrates that can induce energy crashes and surges. Including a moderate amount of these complex carbohydrates in your diet helps ensure that the body has enough energy for yoga practice without feeling heavy or lethargic.

Protein is crucial for muscle repair and growth. Since yoga can sometimes be physically demanding, consuming adequate protein helps repair and strengthen muscles that are worked during practice. Sources of high-quality protein include lean meats, fish, eggs, and, for those who are vegetarian or vegan, beans, lentils, and tofu. These protein sources also contain other valuable nutrients that help support overall health and wellbeing.

Healthy fats are another important component of a yoga-supportive diet. Omega-3 fatty acids, found in fish- like salmon and sardines and in flaxseeds and walnuts, are particularly beneficial. These fats, are not only good for the heart but also help reduce inflammation in the body, which can be beneficial after intense yoga sessions that strain the muscles and joints.

Hydration is another key element that complements the physical practice of yoga. Staying adequately hydrated helps maintain optimal joint lubrication, muscle function, and overall vitality. It also aids in digestion and helps flush toxins from the body, which enhances the detoxifying effects often associated with yoga. Drinking water throughout the day, and especially before and after yoga sessions, ensures that hydration levels are maintained.

Furthermore, incorporating a variety of fruits and vegetables in your diet ensures a high intake of vitamins, minerals, antioxidants, and fibers, which are crucial for maintaining high energy levels, protecting the body against oxidative stress, and ensuring smooth digestive processes. These foods help bolster the immune system, promote healthy skin, and contribute to the overall vitality that is necessary for an effective yoga practice.

For those engaged in more intense yoga practices, incorporating anti-inflammatory foods can help manage and reduce muscle soreness and joint pain. Due to their well-known anti-inflammatory qualities, blueberries, cherries, ginger, and turmeric can all be advantageous dietary additions for yoga practitioners.

Finally, it is important to listen to your body and adjust your dietary needs based on how you feel and the demands of your yoga practice. Everyone's body is different and may require adjustments in macronutrient intake, hydration levels, or specific dietary needs. Maintaining an awareness of how different foods affect your energy levels, mood, and physical wellbeing is crucial.

This mindfulness, developed through yoga, can extend to eating habits, leading to more intuitive eating practices that honor and respond to the body's natural cues.A holistic approach to health that combines yoga with a mindful, balanced diet not only enhances physical health but also supports mental and emotional wellbeing. This synergy between diet and physical activity is key to building a foundation of health that supports a vibrant and fulfilling lifestyle.

Eating for Energy: Nutritional Tips to Complement Your Yoga Practice

Integrating a balanced and thoughtful diet with your yoga practice can significantly boost your energy and enhance your overall wellbeing, ensuring you get the most from your sessions. To sustain energy throughout yoga and aid in recovery and muscle health afterward, it's crucial to focus on nutritional intake that supports both endurance and relaxation.

Starting your day with complex carbohydrates such as whole grains or oats provides a steady release of energy. These foods are essential for keeping you fueled, especially if you practice yoga in the morning or midday. Adding chia seeds to your oatmeal or including quinoa or brown rice in your lunch can maintain stable energy levels during yoga and beyond.

Protein plays a crucial role in muscle repair and growth, which is vital as yoga involves various muscle-strengthening and stretching exercises. Incorporating lean proteins like chicken, fish, tofu, and legumes into your meals not only supports muscle maintenance but also enhances your body's recovery processes after yoga. Options like a grilled salmon salad or a chickpea stew are not only nutritious but also packed with flavors that satisfy.

Healthy fats are another pillar of a diet that complements yoga practice. They provide sustained energy, which is essential for longer sessions, and help with vitamin absorption and inflammation reduction. Including foods like avocados, nuts, seeds, and olive oil in your diet can boost your calorie intake healthily and support your endurance during yoga.

Staying hydrated is equally crucial. Water is central to maintaining optimal physical performance as it aids in nutrient transport, waste removal, and efficient metabolic function. Enhancing your water intake with slices of cucumber or lemon can make hydration more enjoyable while adding some extra nutrients.

Antioxidants are essential for lowering oxidative stress and inflammation in the body, both of which can happen after strenuous yoga sessions. Antioxidant-rich meals like green tea, berries, and leafy vegetables can help reduce muscular soreness and hasten healing. A berry and spinach smoothie post-yoga not only helps with muscle recovery but is also refreshing and revitalizing.

It's important to adjust your diet based on the intensity and nature of your yoga routine. More vigorous sessions might require more proteins for muscle repair, while lighter days might call for simpler meals. Listening to your body's responses to different foods and adjusting your intake accordingly can significantly enhance the benefits of your yoga practice.

Consider also the timing of your meals in relation to your yoga practice. Eating a light meal rich in complex carbohydrates and a bit of protein about an hour before yoga can prevent you from feeling heavy or sluggish during your session. Following up your yoga practice with a balanced meal of proteins and carbohydrates can help replenish energy stores and aid in muscle recovery.

By carefully balancing these nutritional components, you may enhance the overall health advantages of your yoga practice by supporting your mental and emotional wellbeing in addition to your physical health. Each meal becomes an opportunity to nourish your body in a way that supports your physical activities and overall health goals, turning your diet into a fundamental part of your yoga journey.

Anti-inflammatory Foods: Supporting Your Body from Within

Inflammation is the body's natural defense and healing process. On the other hand, persistent inflammation can cause a number of illnesses, including heart disease, arthritis, and even some types of cancer. For individuals engaged in practices like yoga, managing inflammation is crucial not only for enhancing performance but also for speeding up recovery and promoting overall wellbeing. Incorporating anti-inflammatory foods into one's diet can provide the body with the necessary nutrients to combat inflammation effectively.

Antioxidants, omega-3 fatty acids, vitamins, and minerals are abundant in anti-inflammatory diets, and they all function together to lessen inflammation. Such a diet not only supports the physical demands of yoga but also enhances mental clarity and emotional stability.

Omega-3 fatty acids, antioxidants, vitamins, and minerals abound in anti-inflammatory meals, and they all contribute to the reduction of inflammation. A diet like this helps with mental clarity and emotional stability, as well as supporting the physical demands of yoga. These fish not only help lower levels of inflammatory markers in the blood but also contribute to overall heart health and brain function, which are essential for maintaining the focus and dedication required for yoga practice. For vegetarians or those who prefer not to eat fish, flaxseeds, chia seeds, and walnuts are alternative sources of omega-3 fatty acids. These can be easily incorporated into daily meals, such as adding flaxseeds to smoothies or topping salads with walnuts.

Collard greens, spinach, and kale are examples of green leafy vegetables that are a great source of vitamins and minerals, including vitamin E, which has anti-inflammatory qualities. Additionally, a strong supply of antioxidants found in these veggies helps shield the body from oxidative stress, which can cause inflammation. You can be sure that your diet has a range of anti-inflammatory substances that promote general health and muscle recovery when you include a variety of green vegetables in your diet.

Berries such as strawberries, blueberries, raspberries, and blackberries are rich in antioxidants known as flavonoids, which are powerful in reducing inflammation and boosting the body's immune system. These fruits are not only delicious but also versatile and can be enjoyed on their own, in smoothies, or as toppings on cereals and yogurts.

Turmeric, a spice commonly used in Indian cuisine, contains curcumin, a compound with potent anti-inflammatory properties. Curcumin is particularly effective in reducing inflammation in the muscles and joints, making it a beneficial addition for those who practice yoga regularly. You may make a medicinal tea by steeping turmeric leaves in water and then adding them to soups, stews, or smoothies.

Ginger, like turmeric, is another spice that has been shown to have significant anti-inflammatory effects. It works well as tea and in a variety of recipes, like smoothies and stir-fries. Ginger not only helps reduce inflammation but also aids in digestion and nausea, enhancing overall gastrointestinal health.

Nuts are rich in calcium, magnesium, and vitamin E—all of which are necessary for controlling inflammation—especially walnuts and almonds. Nuts are a good source of anti-inflammatory discomfort and stiffness, and they can be especially helpful after long yoga practices.

Extra virgin olive oil is highly valued for its anti-inflammatory and health-promoting properties. It is a mainstay of the Mediterranean diet. Olive oil is a great option for both cooking and salad dressing since it is high in antioxidants and monounsaturated fats, especially oleocanthal, which possesses qualities akin to those of non-steroidal, anti-inflammatory medications.

In the end, studies have demonstrated that a diet high in whole grains, such as brown rice, whole wheat, quinoa, and oats, lowers blood levels of C-reactive protein, a sign of inflammation. In addition to supporting inflammatory health, substituting whole grains for refined carbs can help sustain a consistent energy level.

By integrating these anti-inflammatory foods into your diet, you not only support your body's ability to fight inflammation but also enhance your capability to perform yoga with increased vitality and less discomfort. Such a diet, combined with regular yoga practice, contributes significantly to a holistic health approach, supporting your body from the inside out.

Lifestyle Modifications for Holistic Health

Holistic health encompasses the integration of the mind, body, and spirit within the environment, and achieving it requires attention to various aspects of life, including diet, exercise, sleep hygiene, time management, and stress management. To support holistic health effectively, one must consider making several lifestyle modifications that promote balance and wellbeing across all these areas.

Sleep hygiene is a fundamental pillar of holistic health. Quality sleep affects various functions, including cognitive abilities, emotional balance, and physical health. To improve sleep hygiene, establish a consistent bedtime and wake-up schedule, even on weekends. This regularity reinforces the natural circadian rhythm, helping the body anticipate when to rest and when to awaken. Creating a bedtime routine is also beneficial.

This might involve engaging in relaxing activities like meditation or easy yoga poses, reading a book, or having a warm bath. Make sure the atmosphere where you sleep is restorative by keeping it cold, dark, and quiet. You should also get a good mattress and pillows.

Time management is another critical aspect of living a balanced life. Poor time management can lead to stress, rushed meals, lack of exercise, and shortened sleep, which all detract from holistic health. Begin by prioritizing tasks and setting realistic goals each day. Use tools like calendars or apps to keep track of obligations and commitments. Allocate specific times for work and equal importance to rest and leisure activities. Remember, taking time for yourself is not a luxury but a necessity for maintaining mental and physical health.

A holistic approach to health also heavily relies on nutrition. Consuming a well-balanced diet full of whole grains, fruits, vegetables, lean meats, and healthy fats gives the body the nutrition it needs to perform at its best. Eating mindfully improves the connection with food and reduces overindulgence. Examples of mindful eating techniques include monitoring hunger signs and eating without distractions. To guarantee that you may enjoy a range of nutrients throughout the week and to prevent impulsive bad eating selections at the last minute, think about prepping meals in advance.

All physical and mental wellness depend on physical activity. Frequent exercise lessens anxiety and sadness, enhances sleep quality, and helps control mood. It doesn't have to be strenuous gym activities; regular walking, cycling, or yoga might be beneficial as well. Finding an activity, you love and being consistent are the keys to maintaining a regular workout routine.

Managing stress is essential to preserving overall health. Prolonged stress has been linked to major health problems such as diabetes, heart disease, anxiety, and depression. Stress management techniques, including deep breathing exercises, mindfulness, and meditation, may be incorporated into everyday activities. These practices not only reduce stress but also enhance overall life satisfaction by fostering a greater sense of peace and presence.

In addition to these changes, it's important to foster social connections. Relationships with friends, family, and community are foundational to emotional health and resilience. Social connections can increase emotions of contentment and self-worth while reducing feelings of stress and loneliness. Prioritize spending time with your loved ones, and think about joining clubs or participating in community events that suit your interests.

Modifications to the surroundings might also promote holistic wellness. Organizing your living and working places to clear the clutter and create a peaceful environment might be part of this. Adding natural aspects to your space, such as plants or water features, may make it feel more peaceful. There is evidence that being in a natural environment lowers stress, elevates mood, and improves cognitive performance.

Finally, by encouraging pleasure and life satisfaction, personal development and progress support holistic health. Take part in intellectually and creatively stimulating activities; this may be anything from reading to picking up a new skill to painting or writing; broadening your horizons will help you feel accomplished and fulfilled.

By integrating these lifestyle modifications, you can build a foundation for holistic health that nurtures your physical, mental, and emotional wellbeing, allowing you to lead a balanced and fulfilling life.

Sleep Hygiene: Restorative Sleep for Better Health

However, being crucial for preserving both physical and mental health, sleep hygiene is frequently neglected in our hectic lives. Good sleep hygiene means having both a bedroom environment and daily routines that promote consistent, uninterrupted sleep. Keeping in tune with your body's natural sleep-wake cycle, or circadian rhythms, is one of the most important strategies for achieving restorative sleep.

Creating an environment conducive to sleep begins with optimizing your bedroom. It should be cool, quiet, and dark—excess heat or noise can significantly disturb your sleep. Consider using blackout curtains, eye shades, earplugs, or white noise machines to shield against light and sound. Your mattress and pillows should also be comfortable, supporting your body in a way that does not cause pain or stiffness.

Your pre-sleep activities play a crucial role as well. Before going to bed, you may tell your body it's time to wind down by doing something soothing. This may be doing some light reading, doing a little yoga pose, or going to bed early. Avoiding the displays on computers, cellphones, and televisions is advised because the blue light they generate can disrupt the body's ability to produce melatonin, a hormone that is essential for controlling sleep.

Your sleep quality is also greatly influenced by your diet and level of activity. Sleep disturbances can be avoided by avoiding large meals, coffee, and alcohol close to bedtime. Exercise shortly before bedtime can have the opposite impact of falling asleep more quickly and experiencing deeper sleep, even though exercise during the day can help you do both.

Finally, keeping a regular sleep pattern is essential. Establishing a consistent bedtime and wake-up time each day programs your body's internal clock to anticipate sleep at the same time every night. If you want to prevent a sleep hangover on Monday morning, try to follow your schedule as precisely as possible over the weekends.

Waking up refreshed and alert every morning directly benefits your health, mood, and overall daily performance. Integrating these practices into your life can significantly enhance the quality of your sleep, ensuring you are giving your body the rest it needs to thrive.

Time Management: Balancing Activity and Rest

Time management is crucial for maintaining a healthy balance between activity and rest, ensuring that both are optimized to support overall wellbeing. Effective time management isn't just about being productive; it also involves setting aside enough time for rest and relaxation, which are equally important for maintaining a balanced lifestyle.

Setting work priorities based on significance and urgency is one of the keys to effective time management. This makes it easier to decide what can wait and what requires quick attention. Prioritizing your work can help you better manage your time throughout the day and prevent stress and burnout by preventing important chores from being put off until the last minute. Dividing more complex activities into smaller, more doable phases is also beneficial. This method not only gives the work a clear path to completion but also lessens its intimidating appearance.

Creating a structured daily schedule can significantly enhance your ability to manage time effectively. This includes setting specific times for work, exercise, meals, and rest. A structured schedule helps prevent the day from becoming chaotic and ensures that there's a healthy balance between being productive and taking necessary breaks. It's important to be realistic when planning your day; overloading it can be just as counterproductive as not planning at all.

Incorporating breaks into your day is essential. When you take short pauses, you may relax and rejuvenate, which boosts your productivity when work resumes. Whether it's a short walk, a meditation session, or just stepping away from your work environment, taking breaks can prevent fatigue and enhance cognitive function.

Flexibility is also crucial in time management. While it's important to have a plan, being too rigid can lead to stress. Life is unpredictable, and being able to adapt to changes can reduce anxiety and increase your ability to manage time effectively.

Finally, learning to say no is a powerful tool in time management. Understanding your limits and not overcommitting yourself is crucial for maintaining a healthy balance between activity and rest. Effective time management is crucial for long-term health and pleasure since it guarantees that you are not just productive but also well-rested and stress-free.

CHAPTER 3

CHAIR YOGA EXERCISE

Seated Mountain Pose

The Seated Mountain Pose is a fundamental yoga position adapted for chair yoga, making it accessible and beneficial for individuals at all fitness levels, including those with mobility limitations. This pose serves as a building block for posture and core stability, adapted to be performed while seated to ensure accessibility.

How to Perform Seated Mountain Pose

1. To execute the Seated Mountain Pose, begin by positioning yourself at the front edge of a sturdy chair.
2. Plant your feet firmly on the ground, ensuring they are hip-width apart and your knees form right angles.
3. Rest your hands on your thighs or along the sides of the chair for additional support.
4. Straighten your spine as if a string were pulling you from the crown of your head towards the ceiling, which helps lengthen and align the spine properly. Draw your shoulder blades back gently and down, and engage your core muscles lightly to maintain a strong, upright posture.
5. Focus on maintaining even and deep breaths to help stabilize and energize your pose.

Benefits

The Seated Mountain Pose offers extensive benefits. It is excellent for enhancing posture by strengthening the core and back muscles, essential for supporting the spine. This pose also encourages deeper breathing, which increases oxygen flow and can help improve concentration and reduce stress levels. Regular practice of the Seated Mountain Pose fosters a greater sense of body awareness, or proprioception, which is crucial for balance and overall physical coordination. By reinforcing foundational posture habits, this pose serves as a cornerstone for more advanced practices in chair yoga, contributing to overall mobility and stability.

Chair Cat-Cow Stretch

The Chair Cat-Cow Stretch is a gentle flow between two poses that warms the body and brings flexibility to the spine. It's particularly useful for individuals who spend a lot of time sitting, as it helps to relieve tension in the back and neck.

How to Perform Chair Cat-Cow Stretch

1. To perform the Chair Cat-Cow Stretch, start by sitting on a chair with your feet flat on the floor, hip-width apart.
2. Place your hands on your knees.
3. As you inhale, arch your back, push your belly forward, lift your chest, and look up towards the ceiling, entering the Cow position.
4. As you exhale, round your spine, pull your belly button towards your spine, and tuck your chin to your chest, transitioning into the Cat position.
5. Continue to flow between these two positions with each inhale and exhale, moving slowly and with control.

Benefits

This stretch increases the flexibility of the spine, neck, and shoulders, and helps to lubricate the vertebral discs. It stimulates and massages the abdominal organs, aiding in digestion, and helps to relieve stress and calm the mind. The rhythmic movement also improves coordination and breath awareness.

The Seated Forward Bend is a versatile yoga pose that provides numerous benefits for those looking for a gentle yet effective way to stretch and relax the body. Particularly suitable for individuals who spend long hours sitting, this pose targets the back, hamstrings, and calves, areas that often suffer from prolonged periods of inactivity. Moreover, the Seated Forward Bend is renowned for its ability to reduce stress and promote deep relaxation, making it a valuable exercise for both physical and mental health.

How to Perform Seated Forward Bend

1. Begin by sitting at the edge of your chair with your feet hip-width apart and flat on the floor.

2. Extend your legs slightly, keeping your heels on the ground.

3. Inhale deeply, then exhale as you hinge forward at your hips, reaching your hands towards your feet.

4. Allow your head and neck to relax, and hold onto your shins, ankles, or feet, depending on your flexibility.

5. Maintain a straight spine as you deepen the bend.

Benefits

This pose stretches the entire back of the body, including the spine, hamstrings, and calves. It helps to relieve tension in the spine and improve posture. Additionally, it calms the mind and can reduce symptoms of anxiety and fatigue. By engaging in this forward bend, you allow your body to unwind and release the stress that often accumulates in the lower back and legs due to long periods of sitting.

The Chair Extended Side Angle pose is an excellent exercise for opening the chest and hips while simultaneously strengthening the legs and core. It's a versatile stretch that can be adapted to suit different levels of flexibility, making it accessible for beginners and beneficial for those with more yoga experience. This pose not only improves physical flexibility but also enhances overall body balance and stamina.

How to Perform Chair Extended Side Angle

1. Sit sideways on a chair with your right side facing the backrest.

2. Place your right foot flat on the floor and extend your left leg out to the side, keeping your foot grounded.

3. Rest your right forearm on your right thigh and extend your left arm over your head, reaching towards the right side.

4. Turn your gaze upwards if comfortable.

5. Hold the position, ensuring you feel a stretch but no discomfort. Then, switch sides to maintain balance in your flexibility and strength training.

Benefits

The Chair Extended Side Angle pose offers numerous benefits. It stretches the groin, spine, waist, chest, and shoulders, areas often neglected in daily activities but crucial for overall mobility and comfort. This pose also strengthens the legs, knees, and ankles, promoting muscle endurance and joint health. Additionally, the upward reach and open chest improve respiratory capacity, which can enhance breathing and aid in better oxygen flow throughout the body.

The Seated Spinal Twist is a highly beneficial yoga pose that facilitates increased spinal mobility and improved digestion. This pose is particularly advantageous for alleviating discomfort associated with back pain and stiffness, making it a crucial addition for anyone spending extensive periods seated. The gentle twisting motion not only helps in enhancing flexibility but also supports overall spinal health.

How to Perform Seated Spinal Twist

1. Sit comfortably on your chair with your feet flat on the floor, ensuring your knees are aligned directly above your feet for stability.

2. Place your right hand on the back of the chair and your left hand on your right thigh to aid in facilitating the twist.

3. Inhale deeply to prepare, focusing on elongating your spine upwards to create space between each vertebra.

4. As you exhale, gently twist your torso to the right, using your hands to help deepen the twist gradually. Ensure the movement is smooth and controlled.

5. Hold the position for a few breaths, experiencing the stretch and relaxation it brings. With each inhale, attempt to lengthen the spine further, and with each exhale, ease into the twist a bit more.

Benefits

This pose significantly increases the flexibility of the spine and stimulates the digestive organs, which can aid in detoxification and digestion. It also effectively relieves tension in the back and shoulders, promoting better spinal alignment. The rotational movement involved in the Seated Spinal Twist helps to wring out toxins from the spinal tissues, akin to wringing water from a cloth, which enhances overall circulation and purification within the body.

The Chair Pigeon Pose is a seated modification of the traditional Pigeon Pose, targeting the hips and lower back. It is particularly useful for those with tight hips or lower back pain, offering a way to gently stretch and relieve these common areas of tension.

How to Perform Chair Pigeon Pose

1. Sit upright on a chair with your feet flat on the ground, ensuring that your spine remains aligned and your posture is straight.

2. Carefully lift your right ankle and place it over your left knee, forming a figure four with your legs. This setup is key in targeting the right areas.

3. Keep your right foot flexed throughout the pose. This action helps protect your knee from unnecessary stress and stabilizes the pose.

4. Gradually hinge forward at the hips, bringing your torso closer to your leg. This movement deepens the stretch, so proceed slowly and only to the extent that feels comfortable.

5. Hold this position for several breaths, focusing on relaxing and deepening the stretch with each exhale.

6. After maintaining the pose, gently release and switch sides, ensuring that both hips are equally stretched.

Benefits

The Chair Pigeon Pose is renowned for its ability to deeply stretch the hips, glutes, and lower back. This stretching is crucial for alleviating tension and enhancing flexibility in these areas, often tight due to sedentary lifestyles or certain physical activities.

Seated Leg Lifts are a simple yet effective exercise designed to strengthen the lower abdominal muscles and hip flexors. Ideal for integration into daily routines, this exercise helps enhance core stability and strengthen the lower body without the need for specialized equipment.

How to Perform Seated Leg Lifts

1. Begin by sitting tall on a chair with your feet planted firmly on the ground. Ensure that your spine is straight and your posture is upright to maximize the effectiveness of the exercise.

2. Place your hands on the sides of the chair for added support. This will help stabilize your upper body and allow you to focus on the movement of your legs.

3. Engage your core muscles firmly to provide stability throughout the exercise, protecting your lower back.

4. Slowly lift your right leg, extending it straight out in front of you. Keep the leg elevated and ensure it does not touch the floor to maintain tension in the abdominal muscles.

5. Hold this position for a few seconds to maximize engagement in the core and hip flexor muscles.

6. Gently lower your leg back to the starting position in a controlled manner.

Benefits

Performing Seated Leg Lifts regularly strengthens the lower abdominal muscles, hip flexors, and quadriceps, which are crucial for core stability and overall lower body strength.

Chair Warrior I is a powerful pose that builds strength and stamina while stretching the upper body. It is an excellent pose for improving focus and energy, making it a valuable addition to any seated exercise routine.

How to Perform Chair Warrior I

1. Begin by sitting sideways on a chair, ensuring your right leg is extended behind you and your left foot is flat on the ground. This position allows for a deep stretch and proper alignment of the legs.

2. Align your left knee directly over your left ankle to ensure the leg is at a safe and effective angle for building strength without strain.

3. Raise your arms overhead, keeping them shoulder-width apart to engage the muscles of your arms and upper body fully.

4. Turn your torso to face forward, aligning your chest with your legs. This alignment helps engage your core and provides a full body stretch.

5. Hold the pose for several breaths, focusing on maintaining balance and a strong, upright posture. The duration of holding the pose can increase the intensity and benefits.

6. After holding, gently release and switch sides to ensure balance in muscle strength and flexibility across both sides of the body.

Benefits

Chair Warrior I significantly strengthens the legs and improves overall stability, which is crucial for maintaining mobility and balance. By stretching the chest and shoulders, it helps enhance breathing capacity, contributing to better respiratory health and increased energy levels. The focused nature of the pose also aids in improving concentration and mental clarity, making it a comprehensive exercise for both body and mind.

Chair Warrior II is a dynamic variation that focuses on building strength and flexibility in the legs and hips, while also opening the chest and shoulders. This pose is excellent for enhancing overall body balance and alignment.

How to Perform Chair Warrior II

1. Begin by sitting sideways on a chair, positioning yourself so that your left leg is bent with the foot flat on the floor, and your right leg is extended out to the side, also with the foot flat on the ground. This setup ensures proper alignment and stability.

2. Extend your arms out to the sides at shoulder height, keeping them parallel to the ground. This helps engage your core and upper body muscles effectively.

3. Turn your head to look over your left hand, ensuring your neck remains relaxed and aligned with your spine. This rotation enhances the stretch across your shoulders and neck.

4. Hold this position for several breaths, focusing on maintaining a firm and stable posture. The length of time you hold the pose can intensify the benefits and increase endurance.

5. After holding, carefully switch sides to maintain muscular balance and symmetry in your body.

Benefits

Chair Warrior II is particularly beneficial for strengthening the legs, hips, and core. These areas are crucial for everyday movements and overall physical health. By increasing flexibility in the hips and shoulders, this pose helps to alleviate tension and promote greater range of motion.

The Seated Chair Squat is a dynamic movement that not only helps to strengthen the lower body but also enhances balance and coordination.

How to Perform Seated Chair Squat

1. Begin by sitting on the edge of a chair with your feet flat on the ground and spaced hip-width apart. This starting position ensures that you are stable and prepared to engage the necessary muscles effectively.

2. Engage your core muscles to provide stability throughout the exercise. This is crucial as it helps to protect your lower back and ensures that the upper body remains steady.

3. Lean slightly forward at your hips, which helps to shift your weight and balance. This forward lean is essential for initiating the movement.

4. Press firmly through your heels to lift your hips off the chair. This action activates the quadriceps, hamstrings, and gluteal muscles, which are instrumental in lifting your body.

5. Stand up fully, extending your hips and knees to come to a complete standing position. Ensure your back remains straight and your core engaged.

6. Slowly lower yourself back down to the seated position. This lowering phase is just as important as the ascent because it requires control and muscle engagement to perform smoothly.

Benefits

The Seated Chair Squat is highly effective for strengthening several key muscle groups, including the quadriceps, hamstrings, glutes, and core muscles. These muscles are essential for many daily activities and maintaining good posture.

The Seated Tummy Twist is a gentle yet effective exercise designed to target the oblique muscles. It aids in digestion and enhances spinal flexibility, making it an excellent choice for those looking to improve core strength .

How to Perform Seated Tummy Twist

1. Begin by sitting tall on a chair, ensuring your feet are flat on the floor. This posture helps establish a stable base and proper alignment for the twist.

2. Place your hands on your thighs or the sides of the chair for added stability and control during the exercise.

3. Inhale deeply to lengthen your spine upward, creating space between the vertebrae, which prepares your body for the twisting motion.

4. As you exhale, gently twist your torso to the right. This movement should originate from the lower back, moving upwards; imagine wringing out a towel to engage the correct muscles.

5. Hold the twist for a few breaths, focusing on deepening the stretch with each exhale without straining. This hold allows the muscles to fully engage and the twist to have a more profound effect.

6. Slowly return to the center as you inhale and prepare to repeat the exercise on the left side to ensure balanced muscle development and flexibility.

Benefits

The Seated Tummy Twist offers multiple benefits beyond just strengthening the oblique muscles. By increasing the flexibility of the spine, it helps to maintain a healthy range of motion, crucial for daily activities and preventing injuries.

The Chair Sun Salutation is a series of flowing movements adapted for seated practice, offering the same invigorating and strengthening benefits as the traditional Sun Salutation. This adaptation is particularly beneficial for those who prefer a seated exercise or need a gentler option.

How to Perform Chair Sun Salutation

1. Begin by sitting tall on a chair with your feet firmly planted on the ground, ensuring your spine is straight and your posture is upright.

2. Inhale deeply and raise your arms overhead, bringing your palms together if possible, to fully stretch the upper body.

3. As you exhale, fold forward from the hips, reaching towards your toes. Allow your hands to rest wherever they reach comfortably, which might be your shins, ankles, or feet.

4. Inhale and come halfway up, straightening your back into a flat position. This halfway lift is crucial for preparing the spine for a deeper fold.

5. Exhale and fold forward again, deepening the hinge at your hips and encouraging a greater stretch in the back and hamstrings.

6. On your next inhalation, slowly raise your arms back overhead, lifting your torso and returning to the starting position.

7. Exhale and lower your hands to your thighs, completing one cycle of the Chair Sun Salutation.

Benefits

The Chair Sun Salutation provides a comprehensive workout that warms up the body, enhancing muscle flexibility and strength. It's particularly effective in improving coordination and balance, which are crucial for everyday activities. By synchronizing movements with deep, rhythmic breaths, it promotes better respiratory functions and increases oxygen flow to the brain and other vital organs.

Seated Marching is a straightforward cardiovascular exercise that is effective in increasing heart rate and promoting circulation. It also plays a crucial role in strengthening the lower body, making it a beneficial activity for those seeking a low-impact way to boost their cardiovascular health.

How to Perform Seated Marching

1. Begin by sitting tall on a chair with your feet flat on the ground. Ensure your back is straight and your posture is upright to facilitate proper breathing and alignment.

2. Engage your core to stabilize your upper body and prevent rocking or excess motion as you lift your legs.

3. Lift your right knee towards your chest as high as comfortably possible without straining, then gently lower it back to the starting position.

4. Follow immediately by lifting your left knee in the same manner, creating an alternating marching motion. This rhythmic lifting mimics the natural motion of walking but in a seated position.

5. Use your arms to help maintain balance and establish a steady rhythm. You can swing them alternately as you would when walking briskly, which also adds a slight upper body workout to the motion.

Benefits

Seated Marching is not only simple but also packs a multitude of health benefits. It primarily improves cardiovascular health by increasing the heart rate, which is essential for heart strength and efficiency. The exercise strengthens the hip flexors and thighs, which are crucial for mobility and daily activities.

The Chair Hip Stretch is a gentle yet effective pose designed to target the hip muscles, helping to alleviate tension and improve flexibility.

How to Perform Chair Hip Stretch

1. Start by sitting upright on a chair with your feet flat on the floor, ensuring your spine is straight and your posture is aligned.

2. Carefully cross your right ankle over your left knee, forming a figure four shape with your legs. This position isolates the hip and prepares it for a deep stretch.

3. Keep your right foot flexed throughout the pose. This action helps stabilize the ankle and protect the knee from twisting or undue stress.

4. Gradually hinge forward at the hips, bringing your torso closer to your leg. The depth of the hinge should be determined by your comfort level—aim to feel a stretch, but not pain.

5. Hold this position for several deep breaths, focusing on relaxing into the stretch with each exhale. This will help deepen the stretch without forcing the muscles.

6. After holding, gently release and switch sides to ensure both hips receive equal treatment.

Benefits

The Chair Hip Stretch offers several benefits beyond just relieving hip tension. By stretching the hips, glutes, and lower back, it helps to improve overall flexibility in these crucial areas, which can enhance mobility and ease of movement. This pose also promotes circulation in the lower body, which can help reduce swelling and improve nutrient delivery to the tissues.

Seated Knee Lifts are a straightforward exercise that effectively strengthens the core and hip flexors while also improving coordination and balance. This exercise is particularly beneficial for enhancing functional movements and maintaining lower body strength.

How to Perform Seated Knee Lifts

1. Begin by sitting tall on a chair, ensuring your feet are flat on the floor. This initial posture is crucial for stability and effective execution of the exercise.

2. Engage your core muscles to provide support for your lower back and to stabilize your upper body during the lifts.

3. Gently lift your right knee towards your chest as high as comfortably possible without straining. This movement targets the hip flexors and core.

4. Slowly lower your right knee back to the starting position, controlling the movement to maximize the engagement of your abdominal muscles.

5. Repeat the motion with your left knee, alternating sides to maintain balance in muscle usage and development.

6. Continue to maintain an upright posture throughout the exercise to enhance the benefits and prevent any strain on the back.

Benefits

Seated Knee Lifts are highly effective for strengthening the core muscles and hip flexors, which are crucial for overall stability and movement. The exercise also improves balance and coordination, enhancing the body's ability to perform daily activities more efficiently and safely.

Chair Leg Extensions are a straightforward exercise designed to strengthen the quadriceps and improve leg flexibility, which is crucial for overall lower body strength and stability.

How to Perform Chair Leg Extensions

1. Sit upright on a chair with your feet flat on the floor and your hands resting on the sides of the chair for support. This starting position ensures proper alignment and stability.

2. Slowly extend your right leg straight out in front of you until it is parallel to the floor, keeping your toes pointed upward. This motion engages the quadriceps fully.

3. Hold the position for a few seconds to maximize the engagement of the muscle.

4. Slowly lower your leg back down to the starting position, controlling the movement to engage the muscle throughout the range of motion.

5. Repeat the movement with your left leg, alternating between both legs to maintain balance in muscle development and flexibility.

Benefits

Chair Leg Extensions are beneficial for strengthening the quadriceps, which are key supporters of knee joint health and overall lower limb functionality. This exercise also enhances leg flexibility and core stability, contributing to improved balance and posture. Regular practice can help maintain knee joint health and is particularly beneficial for those looking to improve lower body strength and stability, making it an excellent exercise for enhancing physical capabilities and mobility.

The Seated Hamstring Stretch is an effective pose to stretch the hamstrings and calves, promoting flexibility and reducing tension in the lower back.

How to Perform Seated Hamstring Stretch

1. Sit at the edge of your chair with your feet flat on the floor to ensure a solid base for the stretch.

2. Extend your right leg out in front of you, keeping the heel on the ground and toes pointing upward. This position targets the hamstrings effectively.

3. Inhale to lengthen your spine, creating an erect posture that facilitates a deeper stretch.

4. Exhale as you hinge forward at the hips, reaching towards your toes. Keep your back straight to avoid rounding, which can diminish the stretch's effectiveness.

5. Hold the stretch for several breaths, deepening the stretch with each exhale.

6. Switch legs and repeat the process to ensure balanced flexibility and tension relief in both legs.

Benefits

The Seated Hamstring Stretch provides significant benefits by stretching the hamstrings, calves, and lower back. This alleviates tension and improves flexibility, which can help reduce discomfort from prolonged sitting and enhance overall lower body mobility. Regular stretching of these areas can improve posture and reduce the risk of injuries associated with tight muscles, making this an essential exercise for maintaining flexibility and health.

The Chair Warrior III pose is a modified version of the traditional Warrior III, designed to provide additional support which enhances balance and strengthens the lower body.

How to Perform Chair Warrior III

1. Start by standing behind a chair with your hands resting on the backrest for support. This helps maintain balance during the pose.

2. Shift your weight onto your left leg, keeping a slight bend in the knee to avoid locking it, which can provide better stability and protect the joint.

3. Lean forward, extending your right leg straight back behind you. Aim to form a horizontal line from your fingertips, along your torso, and down to your right heel. This line creates a strong, balanced posture that engages multiple muscle groups.

4. Keep your hands on the back of the chair throughout the pose to help maintain balance and support as you stretch and strengthen your body.

5. Hold the position for a few breaths, focusing on maintaining stability and alignment.

6. Carefully return to the starting position and repeat on the other side, ensuring you balance the exercise by working both sides of your body equally.

Benefits

Chair Warrior III strengthens the legs, back, and core, crucial for overall strength and stability. It also improves balance, an essential aspect of physical fitness that helps prevent falls and injuries. Additionally, this pose stretches the hamstrings and lower back, promoting flexibility and reducing tension in these areas.

The Seated Crescent Moon Pose is designed to stretch the sides of the torso while enhancing spinal flexibility, making it an excellent addition to any chair yoga routine.

How to Perform Seated Crescent Moon Pose

1. Sit upright on a chair with your feet flat on the floor, ensuring your hips and shoulders are aligned and your spine is straight.

2. Extend your arms overhead and interlace your fingers, except for the index fingers, which should point upwards.

3. Inhale deeply to lengthen your spine further, creating space between each vertebra.

4. As you exhale, gently bend to the right, keeping your arms straight and aligned with your ears. This movement targets the left side of your torso, providing a deep stretch.

5. Hold the position for several breaths, deepening the stretch with each exhale without straining.

6. Inhale as you return to the center and prepare to stretch the opposite side to maintain balance in your flexibility and strength.

Benefits

Seated Crescent Moon Pose effectively stretches the sides of the torso, enhancing the flexibility and strength of the core muscles. This flexibility is vital for overall body mobility and health. Additionally, the pose helps in relieving tension in the intercostal muscles, which can enhance lung capacity and promote better breathing.

The Chair Star Pose is a dynamic stretch that effectively opens the chest and strengthens the arms and legs, fostering a sense of expansiveness and vitality.

How to Perform Chair Star Pose

1. Begin by sitting at the edge of your chair, ensuring that your posture is upright and your feet are wide apart and flat on the floor. This base provides stability and room for a proper stretch.

2. Extend your arms out to the sides at shoulder height, aligning them with your legs to create a star shape with your body. This alignment not only engages the arms but also contributes to the overall effectiveness of the pose.

3. Engage your core muscles and lengthen your spine upward. Maintaining this engagement and alignment is crucial for maximizing the benefits of the pose and maintaining balance.

4. Hold this position for several deep breaths, focusing on the stretch across your chest and the engagement of your limbs. Each breath should help you feel more grounded and expansive.

Benefits

The Chair Star Pose offers significant benefits for both physical and mental health. It strengthens the arms, legs, and core, which are essential for overall physical stability and strength. The pose also enhances posture and balance, helping to prevent common issues such as back pain and muscle imbalances. By opening the chest, it improves respiratory function, allowing for deeper breaths that enhance oxygen intake and energy levels.

Seated Bicycle Crunches are an excellent exercise for strengthening the abdominal muscles and enhancing coordination and balance.

How to Perform Seated Bicycle Crunches

1. Start by sitting at the edge of your chair with your feet flat on the floor. This position helps maintain balance during the exercise.

2. Place your hands behind your head to support your neck and maintain alignment.

3. Engage your core muscles tightly to stabilize your upper body and protect your spine.

4. Lift your right knee towards your chest while simultaneously twisting your torso to bring your left elbow towards your right knee. This action creates the "bicycle" motion.

5. Lower your right knee and left elbow back to the starting position.

6. Repeat the movement on the opposite side, lifting your left knee and bringing your right elbow towards it.

7. Continue to alternate sides in a smooth, controlled bicycle pedaling motion.

Benefits

Seated Bicycle Crunches primarily strengthen the abdominal muscles, including the obliques, and hip flexors, enhancing the core's overall stability and strength. This exercise also improves coordination and balance, crucial for daily activities and other physical performances, making it a comprehensive workout for maintaining fitness and agility.

The Chair Floating Stick Pose is a challenging balance exercise that strengthens the core and lower back.

How to Perform Chair Floating Stick Pose

1. Sit at the edge of your chair with your feet flat on the floor, maintaining an upright posture.

2. Lean back slightly while keeping your back straight and your core engaged. This positioning is critical for activating the core muscles throughout the exercise.

3. Lift your legs, extending them straight out in front of you, so they are parallel to the floor. This lifts not only challenges your core muscles but also your leg muscles.

4. Extend your arms forward, parallel to your legs, enhancing the balance challenge of the pose.

5. Hold the position, focusing on maintaining a stable, controlled posture.

Benefits

Chair Floating Stick Pose intensively strengthens the core, legs, and lower back. It improves balance and stability, which are essential for overall body control and coordination, promoting an enhanced ability to perform daily tasks and other physical activities efficiently.

The Seated Eagle Pose is a seated adaptation of the traditional Eagle Pose, targeting the shoulders, upper back, and hips.

How to Perform Seated Eagle Pose

1. Sit upright on a chair with your feet flat on the floor to ensure stability.

2. Cross your right thigh over your left thigh, attempting to wrap your right foot around your left calf if possible. This leg position intensifies the hip stretch.

3. Extend your arms in front of you, crossing your left arm over your right arm at the elbows.

4. Bend your elbows and bring your palms together, or as close as possible, to deepen the stretch across your upper back and shoulders.

5. Hold the position for several breaths, focusing on the stretch and maintaining balance.

6. Release and switch sides, ensuring even stretching and strengthening.

Benefits

Seated Eagle Pose stretches the shoulders, upper back, and hips, which can help relieve tension in these areas. It also improves balance, coordination, and focus, which are beneficial for enhancing concentration and overall mental clarity. Regular practice of this pose can contribute significantly to joint mobility and overall physical harmony.

The Chair Neck Stretch is a gentle exercise designed to alleviate tension in the neck and shoulders, providing relief and increased flexibility.

How to Perform Chair Neck Stretch

1. Begin by sitting upright on a chair with your feet flat on the floor to ensure stability and proper posture.

2. Gently lower your right ear towards your right shoulder, focusing on feeling a stretch along the left side of your neck. This should be a gentle pull, not a forceful stretch.

3. Hold the position for a few breaths, allowing the tension in the neck muscles to release gradually.

4. To deepen the stretch, you can optionally place your right hand on the opposite side of your head and apply gentle pressure to enhance the stretching sensation.

5. After holding for an appropriate duration, carefully bring your head back to the center and repeat the stretch on the other side, lowering your left ear towards your left shoulder.

Benefits

The Chair Neck Stretch is highly beneficial for relieving built-up tension in the neck and shoulders. It improves flexibility in these areas, which can help reduce the discomfort associated with prolonged sitting, driving, or computer use. Regularly performing this stretch can also aid in reducing stress and preventing headaches by promoting better circulation and relaxation in the neck and shoulder regions. This exercise enhances overall neck mobility, making it easier to maintain good posture and alignment throughout the day.

Seated Wrist and Finger Stretches are crucial for maintaining flexibility and preventing strain in the wrists and fingers, especially important for those who frequently engage in typing or manual tasks.

How to Perform Seated Wrist and Finger Stretches

1. Sit upright on a chair with your feet flat on the ground, ensuring a stable and balanced posture.

2. Extend your right arm in front of you with your palm facing up.

3. Use your left hand to gently pull back on the fingers of your right hand, stretching the wrist and forearm. Be careful to apply the force gently to avoid any sharp pain.

4. Hold the stretch for several seconds, feeling the stretch in your wrist and the extension of your forearm.

5. Release the stretch slowly and switch sides, repeating the process with your left hand.

6. For the finger stretches, interlace your fingers and gently press your palms away from your body, extending the stretch across your hands and fingers.

Benefits

Seated Wrist and Finger Stretches offer significant benefits by relieving tension and improving flexibility in the wrists, hands, and fingers. These stretches are particularly beneficial for preventing repetitive strain injuries and can improve hand and wrist function. Regular practice helps maintain dexterity and ease of movement, which is vital for performing daily tasks efficiently and comfortably.

Seated Ankle Rotations are an excellent exercise for improving flexibility and mobility in the ankles, contributing to overall lower body health.

How to Perform Seated Ankle Rotations

1. Sit upright on a chair with your feet flat on the floor to ensure stability and proper posture.

2. Lift your right foot off the ground, keeping your leg bent at the knee.

3. Rotate your right ankle in a clockwise direction for several rotations, focusing on moving through the full range of motion. This helps to engage all the muscles around the ankle.

4. After completing the clockwise rotations, switch to rotating your ankle counterclockwise for an equal number of rotations.

5. Lower your right foot back to the floor and repeat the same process with your left foot, ensuring both ankles receive equal attention and exercise.

Benefits

Seated Ankle Rotations are highly beneficial for enhancing flexibility and mobility in the ankles. By regularly practicing this exercise, you can improve circulation in the lower legs, which helps to prevent stiffness and swelling. This increased mobility and flexibility can reduce the risk of injuries and support overall lower body health, making daily activities like walking and standing more comfortable and efficient. Regular ankle rotations are particularly useful for those who spend long periods sitting, as they promote better blood flow and reduce the likelihood of developing circulation-related issues.

The Chair Low Boat Pose is an effective exercise for strengthening the core and lower back, providing a challenging balance component.

How to Perform Chair Low Boat Pose

1. Begin by sitting at the edge of your chair with your feet flat on the floor, ensuring you have a stable base.

2. Lean back slightly, maintaining a straight back and engaging your core muscles to support the movement.

3. Lift your legs, keeping them straight and parallel to the floor. This position engages the lower abdominal muscles and hip flexors.

4. Extend your arms forward, parallel to your legs, to help maintain balance and further engage the core.

5. Hold the position for several breaths, focusing on maintaining balance and keeping your abdominal muscles engaged.

Benefits

The Chair Low Boat Pose is excellent for strengthening the core, hip flexors, and lower back. It also enhances balance and stability, promoting better overall body control and coordination. This pose is particularly beneficial for improving core strength, which is essential for maintaining good posture and preventing lower back pain.

The Seated Camel Pose is a gentle backbend that effectively stretches the chest, abdomen, and hip flexors, contributing to improved spinal flexibility and posture.

How to Perform Seated Camel Pose

1. Sit upright on a chair with your feet flat on the floor, ensuring your posture is aligned.

2. Place your hands on your lower back with your fingers pointing downward, providing support as you move into the backbend.

3. Inhale deeply to lengthen your spine, creating space between the vertebrae.

4. As you exhale, gently arch your back, lifting your chest and looking up towards the ceiling. This movement opens the chest and stretches the front of the body.

5. Keep your core engaged throughout the pose to support your lower back and prevent strain.

Benefits

The Seated Camel Pose stretches the chest, abdomen, and hip flexors, which can help relieve tension and improve flexibility in these areas. This pose also enhances spinal flexibility, contributing to better posture and potentially alleviating back pain. Additionally, by opening the chest, the Seated Camel Pose promotes better respiratory function, allowing for deeper and more efficient breathing. Regular practice of this pose can lead to improved overall flexibility and a sense of openness in the upper body.

The Chair Core Twist is an effective exercise for strengthening the obliques and increasing spinal flexibility, which also aids in digestion.

How to Perform Chair Core Twist

1. Begin by sitting upright on a chair with your feet flat on the floor, ensuring your posture is straight and your spine is lengthened.

2. Place your right hand on the back of the chair for support and your left hand on your right thigh to assist with the twist.

3. Inhale deeply to lengthen your spine, creating space between the vertebrae.

4. As you exhale, gently twist your torso to the right, using your hands to deepen the twist. Focus on turning from your waist rather than your shoulders.

5. Hold the position for several breaths, allowing the stretch to deepen with each exhale while maintaining a straight spine.

6. Slowly return to the center as you inhale, then repeat the exercise on the other side by placing your left hand on the back of the chair and your right hand on your left thigh.

Benefits

The Chair Core Twist is highly beneficial for strengthening the oblique muscles, which play a crucial role in maintaining core stability and supporting the spine. By increasing spinal flexibility, this exercise helps improve overall mobility and reduce the risk of back pain. Additionally, the twisting motion aids in digestion by massaging the internal organs, promoting better digestive health. Regular practice of the Chair Core Twist can also help relieve tension in the lower back, making it a valuable exercise for enhancing both physical health and overall well-being.

The Seated Oblique Bend is an effective exercise that stretches the sides of the torso and strengthens the oblique muscles, enhancing overall flexibility.

How to Perform Seated Oblique Bend

1. Sit upright on a chair with your feet flat on the floor to ensure a stable base and proper posture.

2. Extend your right arm overhead, reaching towards the ceiling.

3. Lean to the left side, feeling a stretch along your right side from your hip up through your ribcage. Ensure the movement is smooth and controlled to avoid any strain.

4. Hold the stretch for a few breaths, allowing the muscles to relax and lengthen with each exhale.

5. Return to the center and switch sides, extending your left arm overhead and leaning to the right.

Benefits

The Seated Oblique Bend provides a deep stretch to the sides of the torso and strengthens the oblique muscles, which are crucial for core stability and movement. This exercise improves overall flexibility and helps to relieve tension in the ribcage and lower back.

By regularly practicing this pose, you can promote better posture and mobility, making it easier to perform daily activities and reducing the risk of injury.

The Chair Tree Pose is a seated adaptation of the traditional Tree Pose, focusing on balance and strength while providing support for those with mobility challenges.

How to Perform Chair Tree Pose

1. Sit upright on a chair with your feet flat on the floor, ensuring your posture is aligned and your spine is straight.

2. Lift your right foot and place it on the inside of your left thigh or shin, depending on your flexibility and comfort level.

3. Press your palms together in front of your chest in a prayer position, helping to maintain balance and engage your core.

4. Hold the pose for several breaths, concentrating on maintaining your balance and keeping your spine lengthened.

5. Carefully lower your right foot back to the floor and repeat the pose on the other side, lifting your left foot and placing it on the inside of your right thigh or shin.

Benefits

The Chair Tree Pose offers numerous benefits, including strengthening the legs and improving balance, which are essential for overall stability and mobility. This pose also enhances concentration as it requires focus to maintain balance. Additionally, it helps to open the hips and stretch the inner thighs, promoting greater flexibility and reducing tension in these areas. The Chair Tree Pose is particularly beneficial for individuals with mobility challenges, providing a supportive way to practice balance and strength exercises safely.

Seated March with Arm Swing is an invigorating exercise that combines lower and upper body movements to enhance coordination and increase cardiovascular health.

How to Perform Seated March with Arm Swing

1. Begin by sitting upright on a chair with your feet flat on the floor, ensuring your spine is straight for proper posture.

2. Start by lifting your right knee towards your chest while simultaneously swinging your left arm forward and the right arm back. This opposite arm and leg movement helps engage the core and improves balance.

3. Lower your right leg and switch to the left leg, lifting your left knee while swinging your right arm forward and the left arm back. The continuous movement mimics a natural walking motion.

4. Keep the movements controlled and rhythmic, focusing on the coordination between your arms and legs.

5. Continue alternating the legs and arms in a marching motion, maintaining a steady pace to keep your heart rate up.

Benefits

Seated March with Arm Swing is a comprehensive exercise that stimulates not only the muscles but also the cardiovascular system. By engaging both the arms and legs in vigorous movements, it helps to improve overall coordination and body balance. This exercise also increases heart rate, promoting better blood circulation and enhancing cardiovascular health. The dynamic arm swings added to the marching motion help to tone the arm muscles and increase upper body mobility.

The Chair Glute Bridge is an effective exercise that focuses on strengthening the glutes and lower back, crucial for enhancing core stability and overall posture.

How to Perform Chair Glute Bridge

1. Start by sitting at the edge of your chair with your feet flat on the floor, placed hip-width apart. This position provides the necessary balance and support for the exercise.

2. Place your hands on the seat beside you for additional stability.

3. Lean back slightly, maintaining a slight angle in your upper body to prepare for the lift.

4. Engage your core and glutes as you lift your hips off the chair, aiming to create a straight line from your knees to your shoulders. Ensure your glutes are tightly squeezed to maximize the exercise's effectiveness.

5. Hold this lifted position for a few seconds, focusing on maintaining tightness in your core and glutes to support your lower back.

6. Slowly lower your hips back down to the chair, controlling the movement to maximize the strengthening effect on the descent.

Benefits

The Chair Glute Bridge is particularly beneficial for strengthening the glutes, lower back, and core muscles. By enhancing the strength in these areas, the exercise improves hip mobility and stability, which are essential for a variety of daily activities and athletic movements. Regular practice of the Chair Glute Bridge can also help alleviate lower back pain by strengthening the supporting muscles around the spine, providing better structural support and reducing strain.

Seated Chair Tappers are a straightforward exercise that effectively improves coordination and leg strength.

How to Perform Seated Chair Tappers

1. Begin by sitting upright on a chair with your feet flat on the ground. Ensure your back is straight and your posture is aligned for optimal performance.

2. Start the exercise by lifting your right foot slightly and tapping your toes on the ground.

3. Quickly switch to your left foot, lifting it and tapping the toes on the ground.

4. Continue alternating between your right and left foot in a rhythmic pattern, maintaining a steady and controlled pace.

5. Aim to continue this tapping motion for several minutes, focusing on the precision and speed of each tap to enhance coordination.

Benefits

Seated Chair Tappers not only improve coordination but also strengthen the leg muscles, contributing to overall lower body strength. This exercise enhances cardiovascular health by keeping the heart rate up during the rhythmic motion. Additionally, it promotes better circulation in the lower body, which can help prevent stiffness and improve mobility.

The Chair Reverse Plank is a challenging exercise that targets multiple muscle groups including the core, arms, and shoulders, and offers a stretch for the front body.

How to Perform Chair Reverse Plank

1. Sit at the edge of your chair with your feet flat on the floor and your hands placed on the seat beside your hips, fingers pointing forward.

2. Engage your core muscles firmly to prepare for the lift.

3. Press down through your hands and lift your hips off the chair, extending your legs out in front of you.

4. Aim to form a straight line from your head to your heels, engaging your glutes and shoulders to maintain the position.

5. Hold this reverse plank for several breaths, focusing on maintaining a strong and stable posture.

6. Carefully lower your hips back to the chair to release the pose.

Benefits

The Chair Reverse Plank significantly strengthens the core, arms, and shoulders. This exercise not only improves muscle tone but also stretches the chest and the front of the body, promoting flexibility. Additionally, the Chair Reverse Plank enhances balance and stability, which can benefit overall physical performance and posture. Regular practice of this pose can contribute to a stronger, more balanced physique.

Seated Toe Taps are an easy yet effective exercise designed to enhance foot and ankle mobility and coordination.

How to Perform Seated Toe Taps

1. Begin by sitting upright on a chair with your feet flat on the floor. Ensure your back is straight to maintain good posture throughout the exercise.

2. Start by lifting your right foot slightly off the ground and then tap your toes back onto the floor.

3. Quickly switch to your left foot, lifting it and tapping the toes on the ground.

4. Continue this motion, alternating between your right and left foot in a rhythmic pattern. The movement should be controlled and consistent to maximize the benefits.

5. Keep the exercise going for several minutes, gradually increasing the speed as your coordination improves.

Benefits

Seated Toe Taps are beneficial for enhancing mobility in the feet and ankles, making them more flexible and less prone to injuries. The rhythmic and repetitive nature of the exercise helps improve coordination, making everyday movements that involve footwork easier and more efficient. Additionally, this exercise stimulates circulation in the lower extremities, which is crucial for vascular health and can help prevent issues related to poor blood flow. Regularly integrating Seated Toe Taps into your routine can contribute significantly to maintaining lower extremity health, especially for individuals who spend a lot of time seated.

Seated Arm Circles are a gentle exercise designed to increase shoulder flexibility and strength, ideal for improving upper body mobility.

How to Perform Seated Arm Circles

1. Start by sitting upright on a chair with your feet flat on the floor, ensuring your posture is aligned and stable.

2. Extend your arms out to the sides at shoulder height, making sure your arms are parallel to the floor.

3. Begin to make small circles with your arms, focusing on keeping the movement smooth and controlled.

4. Gradually increase the size of the circles to further challenge your shoulder flexibility and arm strength.

5. After about a minute, reverse the direction of the circles, continuing the exercise to ensure balanced muscle engagement.

Benefits

Seated Arm Circles effectively increase shoulder flexibility and strengthen the muscles in the arms, enhancing overall upper body mobility. This exercise also improves coordination, which can benefit daily activities that require arm movement. Regular practice promotes better posture and alignment, as the movements help to tone the shoulder muscles and support the correct positioning of the spine.

Chair Push-ups are a modified version of traditional push-ups that provide an accessible yet effective upper body workout.

How to Perform Chair Push-ups

1. Stand behind a chair and place your hands on the seat, ensuring they are shoulder-width apart for proper support.

2. Step back until your body forms a straight line from your head to your heels, establishing a strong plank position.

3. Lower your chest towards the chair while keeping your elbows close to your body to maximize the engagement of your chest and arm muscles.

4. Push back up to the starting position, using your arms and chest to lift your body away from the chair.

5. Repeat the movement, maintaining form and alignment throughout each repetition.

Benefits

Chair Push-ups strengthen the chest, shoulders, triceps, and core, contributing to improved upper body strength and stability. This exercise is particularly beneficial for enhancing muscle tone and endurance in the arms and chest, and it also promotes better posture by strengthening the core muscles that support spinal alignment.

Seated Scissor Kicks are a dynamic exercise that targets the lower abdominal muscles and improves coordination, making them ideal for enhancing core stability.

How to Perform Seated Scissor Kicks

1. Sit at the edge of your chair with your feet flat on the floor to ensure a stable starting position.

2. Lean back slightly, using your arms to hold onto the sides of the chair for support. This posture helps engage your core throughout the exercise.

3. Lift your legs off the floor and begin to alternately cross them over each other in a scissor-like motion. The movement should be controlled and deliberate to maximize engagement of the abdominal muscles.

4. Continue this motion for several minutes, maintaining a steady pace and keeping your core engaged to support the lower back.

Benefits

Seated Scissor Kicks effectively strengthen the lower abdominal muscles, which are crucial for overall core stability. This exercise also improves coordination, helping to synchronize movements between different parts of the body. Regular practice can enhance core strength, making it easier to perform daily activities and reducing the risk of back injuries.

Chair Burpees offer a modified version of the traditional burpee to improve cardiovascular health, strength, and coordination while being accessible for those who need a less intense option.

How to Perform Chair Burpees

1. Begin by sitting at the edge of your chair with your feet flat on the floor, preparing for movement.

2. Place your hands on the seat of the chair and use them to lift your hips off the chair, extending your legs behind you into a plank position supported by the chair.

3. Perform a push-up, maintaining a straight line from your head to your heels to engage the upper body and core fully.

4. Jump your feet back towards the chair, coming into a squat position.

5. Stand up and lift your hands overhead, adding an explosive movement to the exercise.

6. Return to the starting seated position and repeat the sequence for several repetitions.

Benefits

Chair Burpees provide a full-body workout that enhances cardiovascular health and increases strength and coordination. The exercise improves upper and lower body strength and boosts heart rate, contributing to better cardiovascular fitness. Additionally, it enhances balance and stability, which are crucial for performing everyday activities safely and effectively. This version of burpees is especially beneficial for those looking to maintain fitness levels with exercises that are adaptable to their needs.

Dear Readers,

Thank you for allowing us to be a part of your wellness journey. If you have a moment, please consider sharing your experiences so far by leaving a review on Amazon. Your insights can help others feel motivated and supported as they embark on or continue their own journeys in yoga.

How You Can Share Your Review

Through Amazon.com:

1. Go to the Amazon page where you found my book.

2. Navigate to the 'Customer Reviews' section.

3. Click on 'Write a customer review' to share your valuable insights.

Instant QR Code Access: Simply scan the QR code below with your smartphone to be directed to the Amazon review section.

CHAPTER 4

BONUS CHAPTER

One-Week Meal Plan with healthy and tasty recipes

Creating a one-week meal plan that focuses on health and weight loss doesn't have to involve complicated recipes or unavailable ingredients. Instead, it can be based on simple, nutritious meals that are easy to prepare and enjoyable to eat. This meal plan includes a variety of foods that promote weight loss by incorporating high-fiber, low-calorie ingredients that are rich in nutrients.

Day 1

Breakfast: Start your day with a smoothie made from spinach, a small banana, , a handful of frozen berries, a tablespoon of flaxseeds, and a cup of unsweetened almond milk. This smoothie is rich in fiber and antioxidants.

Lunch: Prepare a quinoa salad with chopped cucumber, cherry tomatoes, red onion, a sprinkle of feta cheese, and a dressing of lemon juice and olive oil. Quinoa is high in protein and fiber, which are essential for weight loss.

Dinner: Make a stir-fried chicken with a mix of bell peppers, broccoli, and snap peas, seasoned with garlic, ginger, and a touch of soy sauce. Serve this with a side of brown rice.

Breakfast: Oatmeal made with skim milk, topped with sliced almonds and apple slices. Add a dash of cinnamon for flavor and its blood sugar-regulating benefits.

Lunch: A whole-grain wrap filled with mixed greens, sliced turkey breast, avocado, and a light spread of mustard. Turkey is a great source of lean protein that helps keep you feeling full.

Dinner: Baked salmon with a side of roasted Brussels sprouts and sweet potatoes. Salmon is loaded with omega-3 fatty acids, which are good for heart health.

Day 3:

Breakfast: Greek yogurt topped with a mix of fresh berries and a sprinkle of granola for crunch. Greek yogurt is a fantastic source of protein and probiotics.

Lunch: Lentil soup with a variety of vegetables like carrots, zucchini, and spinach. Lentils are fiber-rich and provide a good amount of plant-based protein.

Dinner: Grilled lean steak with a side of asparagus and quinoa. Choose a lean cut of beef for lower fat content.

Day 4:

Breakfast: A smoothie made from kale, pineapple, cucumber, and coconut water. This combination is hydrating and packed with nutrients.

Lunch: Chickpea salad with red onion, cherry tomatoes, cucumber, and a dressing made from olive oil and balsamic vinegar. Chickpeas are an excellent source of fiber and protein.

Dinner: Turkey meatballs served with spaghetti squash and a homemade tomato sauce. This meal is low in carbohydrates and high in protein.

Breakfast: Scrambled eggs with spinach and mushrooms. Eggs are a high-quality protein source and highly satiating.

Lunch: Grilled vegetable and hummus wrap using whole grain tortillas. The vegetables provide nutrients and fiber, while hummus provides a creamy texture and additional protein.

Dinner: Baked cod with a crust of crushed almonds, served with a side of steamed green beans and carrots.

Day 6:

Breakfast: Chia pudding made by soaking chia seeds in almond milk overnight, topped with kiwi and coconut flakes. Chia seeds are rich in omega-3 fatty acids and fiber.

Lunch: Quinoa and black bean stuffed peppers. This meal is not only visually appealing but also packed with fiber and protein.

Dinner: Grilled chicken breast served with a kale and avocado salad. Add pumpkin seeds for extra crunch and zinc.

Day 7:

Breakfast: Overnight oats prepared with rolled oats, chia seeds, skim milk, and topped with fresh mango slices.

Lunch: Beetroot and goat cheese arugula salad, with walnuts and a simple dressing of olive oil and lemon juice. Beets are high in immune-boosting vitamins and minerals.

Dinner: Stir-fried tofu with a variety of colorful vegetables such as bell peppers, snow peas, and bok choy in a light soy sauce and sesame oil dressing. Tofu is a great source of protein and an excellent meat alternative.

This meal plan provides balanced meals that focus on vegetables, lean proteins, and whole grains while incorporating healthy fats and dairy. Each meal is designed to be simple to prepare, ensuring that maintaining a healthy diet is achievable and enjoyable. By planning meals that are nutrient-dense and portion-controlled, weight loss becomes a natural and satisfying process.

31-Day Challenge: 10 Minutes Daily Workouts

Embarking on a 31-day fitness challenge is an excellent way to commit to your health and fitness, particularly if you're pressed for time. This plan is designed to fit into just 10 minutes each day, ensuring it's manageable for everyone, regardless of their busy schedules. Over the course of the month, the intensity and variety of exercises will gradually increase, allowing your body to adapt and improve without being overwhelmed.

Week 1: Foundation and Mobility

The first week is all about laying a solid foundation and enhancing mobility. Start with basic exercises that focus on large muscle groups and core stability.

- **Day 1:** Start with a simple 5-minute warm-up consisting of marching in place and arm circles, followed by 5 minutes of basic bodyweight exercises: 10 squats, 10 push-ups (knees or full), and 10 sit-ups.

- **Day 2:** Focus on leg strength with lunges. Alternate legs for a total of 5 minutes, then spend the next 5 minutes doing planks, holding for 30 seconds on and 30 seconds off.

- **Day 3:** Introduce dynamic stretches such as leg swings and arm swings for 5 minutes, followed by a 5-minute session of jumping jacks to get the heart rate up.

- **Day 4:** Repeat the routine from Day 1, aiming to increase the number of squats, push-ups, and sit-ups in the same time frame.

- **Day 5:** Add side planks to your routine, holding each side for 30 seconds, alternating for 5 minutes. Follow this with 5 minutes of gentle yoga poses focusing on flexibility.

- **Day 6:** Implement a mini circuit: 2 minutes each of lunges, sit-ups, push-ups, and a cool down with stretching.

- **Day 7:** Active rest day. Spend 10 minutes doing a walking meditation or a gentle stretching routine to help the body recover.

Week 2: Building Intensity

In the second week, you'll start to increase the intensity of your workouts, adding more time under tension and more complex movements.

- **Day 8:** Introduce interval training. Sprint for 30 seconds, then walk for 30 seconds. Repeat for 10 minutes.

- **Day 9:** Circuit training with 1 minute each: squats, push-ups, burpees, and sit-ups, followed by 1 minute of stretching.

- **Day 10:** Add resistance with household items like water bottles. Perform bicep curls, tricep dips, and shoulder presses.

- **Day 11:** Focus on core strength. Perform Russian twists, bicycle crunches, and leg raises for 3 minutes each.

- **Day 12:** Cardio blast with high knees, butt kicks, and mock jumping rope for 3 minutes each.

- **Day 13:** Repeat the circuit from Day 9 but try to add more reps within each 1-minute period.

- **Day 14:** Another active rest day, this time including a foam rolling session or a longer yoga sequence to stretch out tight muscles.

Week 3: Advancement and Challenge

During the third week, further challenge yourself by adding more advanced exercises and increasing the duration of each.

- **Day 15:** Start with a Tabata workout: 20 seconds of intense activity followed by 10 seconds of rest. Choose four exercises like burpees, mountain climbers, squats, and plank jacks. Cycle through twice.

- **Day 16:** Incorporate a Pilates routine focusing on core and flexibility for 10 straight minutes.

- **Day 17:** Add a low-impact strength day using resistance bands for squats, chest presses, and rows.

- **Day 18:** Agility training: set up a small agility ladder or mark areas on the ground to hop in and out quickly for 10 minutes.

- **Day 19:** Increase the Tabata to four cycles, adding exercises like high knees and push-ups.

- **Day 20:** Active recovery with a focus on balance and stretching. Perform single-leg stands, gentle lunges, and extensive stretching.

- **Day 21:** Rest or very gentle yoga focused on deep breathing and slow movements.

Week 4: Peak and Maintenance

The final week is about peaking your performance and starting to think about how to maintain these fitness levels.

- **Day 22:** Challenge yourself with a 10-minute continuous bodyweight workout. See how many rounds you can do of 10 push-ups, 15 squats, and 20 sit-ups.

- **Day 23:** High-intensity interval training (HIIT) for 10 minutes. Choose three high-intensity exercises and perform each for one minute with 30 seconds of rest in between. Repeat twice.

- **Day 24:** Incorporate a kickboxing routine focusing on punches and kicks to boost cardiovascular health and improve coordination.

- **Day 25:** Yoga flow session, integrating strength poses like Warrior III and balances like Tree Pose to enhance strength and flexibility.

- **Day 26:** Full body circuit with minimal rest. Include exercises like lunges, plank holds, squat jumps, and arm circles.

- **Day 27:** Sprint intervals for 10 minutes, aiming to increase the speed or duration of each sprint slightly.

- **Day 28:** Gentle recovery day focusing on stretching and mindfulness to prepare for the final push.

Final Days: Reflection and Forward Planning

- **Day 29:** Perform a personal best challenge. Pick three exercises from the month that you felt were most beneficial and see how many you can do in 10 minutes.

- **Day 30:** Slow-paced, meditative yoga to reflect on the month and focus on deep stretching.

- **Day 31:** Plan a 10-minute dance celebration, choosing your favorite upbeat music and just moving freely to celebrate your dedication and progress over the month.

This 31-day challenge not only helps improve physical fitness but also enhances mental toughness and perseverance. Each day builds on the last, creating a routine that is challenging yet achievable, pushing you towards better health and fitness in manageable increments.

Guided Meditation for Stress Reduction

Guided meditation for stress reduction is a powerful tool that can transform your mental and emotional state, bringing about a sense of peace and clarity. Engaging in regular meditation can help you manage stress more effectively, improve your focus, and promote overall well-being. Here, I'll walk you through a few easy meditation methods that you may use to improve your everyday routine and promote calmness and focus.

Begin by finding a quiet, comfortable space where you won't be disturbed. You can sit in a chair with your feet flat on the floor, cross-legged on the floor, or lie down if that's more comfortable. The key is to find a position where you can be still and relaxed without discomfort. Close your eyes and take a few deep breaths, inhaling through your nose and exhaling through your mouth, allowing your body to begin relaxing with each breath.

Basic Breath Awareness Meditation

This technique focuses on the breath as a point of concentration, helping to anchor your mind in the present moment.

To begin, take a few deep breaths to center yourself. After then, let your breathing settle back into its regular pattern. As air enters and exits your nose, pay attention to how it feels. With every breath in and breath out, feel your belly and chest rise and fall. Refocus your attention on your breathing softly and without passing judgment whenever your thoughts stray. As you get more accustomed to the method, progressively extend the time you spend practicing for a total of five to 10 minutes breath awareness meditation eases mental tension, lowers anxiety, and improves your capacity for sustained attention in day-to-day activities.

Body Scan Meditation

This method entails fostering relaxation, lowering physical tension, and raising awareness of various body areas to start, take a few seconds to center yourself by concentrating on your breath. Then, bring your attention to your feet. Notice any sensations—tingling, warmth, or pressure. Slowly move your attention up to your ankles, calves, knees, and thighs, observing any feelings in each area. Continue this process, moving up through your body—hips, lower back, abdomen, chest, upper back, shoulders, arms, hands, neck, and head. Spend a few moments on each part, noticing sensations and allowing any tension to melt away with each exhale. This meditation can take anywhere from 10 to 20 minutes, depending on how long you spend on each body part.

The body scan meditation can help you develop a deeper connection with your body, promote relaxation, and improve your ability to manage stress.

Loving-Kindness Meditation

This technique focuses on cultivating feelings of compassion and love towards yourself and others.

Begin by taking a few deep breaths and settling into your position. Bring to mind a person or pet for whom you have strong, positive feelings. Visualize them clearly and hold them in your heart. Repeat silently wishes like "may you live with ease, may you be happy, may you be healthy, may you be safe." Give yourself permission to really experience these wishes. After a little while, focus on yourself and say these affirmations to yourself: "May I be happy, may I be healthy, may I be safe, may I live with ease." Last but not least, repeat the lines and radiate your loving-kindness toward friends, family, and eventually all living things as you broaden your focus to include them.

Loving-kindness meditation can enhance your sense of connection, reduce feelings of anger and resentment, and increase your overall sense of well-being.

Visualization Meditation

This method creates a peaceful and upbeat mental environment by utilizing the power of imagination. To begin, close your eyes and focus yourself by taking several deep breaths. Visualize a peaceful place—a beach, a forest, a mountain top, or any place where you feel safe and relaxed. Engage all your senses: imagine the sounds, smells, colors, and sensations associated with this place. Spend a few minutes exploring this environment in your mind, allowing yourself to feel completely immersed in the tranquility of your visualization. Remind yourself to return to the serene vision whenever your thoughts stray. For ten to fifteen minutes, keep up this technique.

Visualization meditation can provide a mental escape from the demands of daily life while also potentially lowering stress and elevating mood.

Mindfulness Meditation

This method, which entails paying attention to the here and now without passing judgment, promotes focus and serenity. Begin by taking a few deep breaths to center yourself. Focus your attention on your breath, the sensations in your body, or the sounds around you. The goal is not to empty your mind but to observe your thoughts and feelings without getting caught up in them. Gently return your attention to the focal point you have selected whenever your thoughts stray from it. Spend five to ten minutes practicing this, and as you get more comfortable, progressively extend the duration. You may become more focused, more adept at managing stress, and more aware of the present moment overall by practicing mindfulness meditation.

Progressive Muscle Relaxation

Through the tensing and releasing of various muscle groups, this approach facilitates physical relaxation and alleviates tension.

Begin by sitting or lying down comfortably. Take a few deep breaths to center yourself. Start with your feet, tensing the muscles as much as you can for five seconds, then releasing the tension completely. Notice the difference between tension and relaxation. Repeat the technique on your calves, thighs, buttocks, belly, chest, arms, hands, neck, and face. Take a few seconds to relish the sensation of calm that permeates your entire body.

Progressive muscle relaxation can lessen anxiety, enhance the quality of sleep, and alleviate physical stress.

Counting Meditation

This technique uses counting to help focus the mind and create a sense of calm.

Sit comfortably and close your eyes. Begin to count your breaths silently: inhale (one), exhale (two), inhale (three), and so on up to ten. Then start again from one. If your mind wanders, gently bring your focus back to the breath and start counting again. Practice this for five to ten minutes, gradually increasing the time as you become more comfortable.

Counting meditation helps to quiet the mind, reduce stress, and improve concentration.

Walking Meditation

This technique combines movement with mindfulness, making it a great option for those who find sitting meditation challenging.

Look for a peaceful area where you may take short strolls. Take a few deep breaths, stand motionless, and focus on becoming aware of your body. Begin to walk slowly, focusing on the sensation of your feet touching the ground. Pay attention to the movements of your legs, the shift of your weight, and your breath. When you reach the end of your path, pause, take a breath, and turn around. Continue walking mindfully for 10 to 15 minutes.

Walking meditation can help increase mindfulness, reduce stress, and improve your connection with your body.

Gratitude Meditation

This method focuses on developing an attitude of thankfulness, which can enhance happiness and general well-being.

Close your eyes and take a comfortable seat. Breathe deeply for a few moments to help you center. Think of people, objects, or facets of your life for which you are thankful. Feel your heart filled with thankfulness as you visualize each one. Say "thank you" quietly for everything. Take a moment to consider all of the blessings in your life and the gratitude they bring.

Gratitude meditation can help improve your mood, increase happiness, and reduce stress.

By incorporating these guided meditation techniques into your daily routine, you can create a powerful practice that helps manage stress, improve mental clarity, and enhance overall well-being. As you get more accustomed to it, progressively extend the duration each day from a few minutes at first. Try to include meditation on a daily basis; consistency is the key. Your capacity to manage stress, concentrate, and preserve inner serenity will probably show noticeable gains over time.

Safety Tips for Chair Yoga

People of all ages and skill levels may benefit greatly from chair yoga, but it's especially beneficial for people who have restricted mobility, balance problems, or are new to exercising. But like with any physical exercise, it's crucial to perform chair yoga properly to avoid injuries and guarantee a good experience. When doing chair yoga, keep these vital safety precautions in mind.

First and foremost, it is crucial to choose the right chair. A stable, sturdy chair without wheels is ideal. Make sure the chair is on a flat surface to prevent it from tipping over. If possible, use a chair with armrests and a straight back for additional support. Avoid chairs that are too soft or have cushions that might cause you to sink in and lose stability.

Proper alignment is key to preventing injuries in chair yoga. Always sit with your feet flat on the floor, hip-width apart, and your knees aligned over your ankles. Your back should be straight, and your shoulders should be relaxed away from your ears. To maintain your spine, contract your core muscles and resist the need to sag or tilt to one side. Sustaining proper posture enhances the protective effects on your back and boosts the efficiency of the workouts.

Listen to your body and respect its limits. Yoga should never cause pain. If you experience any discomfort or pain, ease out of the pose and rest. It is normal to feel a stretch, but sharp pain is a signal that you need to stop. Modify poses to suit your comfort level, and do not force your body into any position. Overstretching can lead to injuries, so always work within your range of motion.

Warm-up is essential before starting your chair yoga session. Gentle movements like shoulder rolls, neck stretches, and ankle rotations can help prepare your muscles and joints for more intense stretches. Warming up increases blood flow to the muscles and reduces the risk of injury. Take at least five to ten minutes to perform warm-up exercises before moving on to the main yoga poses.

A key component of yoga that improves posture efficacy and reduces injury risk is breathing. During your practice, pay close attention to your deep, steady breathing. Breathe in via your nose, opening your abdomen, and then gently release the air through your mouth. Your practice will be safer and more pleasurable if you can better focus and relax by coordinating your breath with your movements.

When performing chair yoga, move slowly and mindfully. Rapid or jerky movements can lead to strains or sprains. Transition smoothly between poses, paying attention to how your body feels. This mindfulness helps you stay aware of your body's limits and prevents overexertion. If you feel tired or unsteady, take a break and resume when you feel ready.

Using props can enhance your chair yoga practice and provide additional support. Yoga straps, blocks, and cushions can help you maintain proper alignment and make poses more accessible. For example, using a strap to reach your feet in a forward bend can prevent overstretching and reduce strain on your back. Place a cushion or rolled towel behind your lower back for extra lumbar support if needed.

It's critical to stay hydrated, particularly while training in a heated setting. Throughout your session, take little sips from the bottle of water that you keep close by. By supporting muscular function and preserving your energy levels, staying hydrated lowers your chance of cramping and other dehydration-related problems.

It is strongly advised that you speak with a healthcare provider before beginning a chair yoga program, particularly if you have any underlying medical issues or concerns. They can ensure that your practice is safe and useful by offering customized guidance and adaptations based on your health situation.

It is also important to pay attention to the environment in which you practice chair yoga. Ensure that the area around your chair is clear of obstacles and clutter to prevent tripping or falling. Adequate lighting is essential to see your surroundings clearly, and practicing in a quiet space can help you focus better and reduce distractions.

Regular practice is key to gaining the benefits of chair yoga, but it is equally important to allow your body to rest and recover. Avoid practicing the same poses every day to prevent overuse injuries. Incorporate variety into your routine and listen to your body's signals to determine when it needs a break.

Incorporating relaxation techniques at the end of your chair yoga session can further enhance safety and well-being. Spend a few minutes in a comfortable seated position, focusing on your breath and allowing your body to relax completely. This practice can help reduce muscle tension and promote a sense of calm.

For those with balance issues, it may be helpful to practice chair yoga near a wall or sturdy surface for additional support. This can provide an extra layer of safety, especially when performing standing poses or transitions that require balance.

Being mindful of any medical devices or aids you may use, such as walkers or hearing aids, is also important. Ensure they are positioned safely and do not interfere with your movements. If necessary, adjust your practice to accommodate these devices.

Ultimately, the keys to a successful and safe chair yoga practice are perseverance and consistency. Proceed at your own speed and acknowledge little accomplishments along the route. Developing strength, flexibility, and balance takes time; yoga is a journey, not a sprint.

By following these safety tips, you can enjoy the numerous benefits of chair yoga while minimizing the risk of injury. This practice can improve your physical health, enhance mental clarity, and promote overall well-being. Remember to always listen to your body, move mindfully, and prioritize safety in every session. With regular practice and attention to safety, chair yoga can become a valuable and enjoyable part of your wellness routine.

Posture Correction Advice

Good posture is essential not only for overall health but also to maximize the benefits of chair yoga. Proper alignment ensures that you are engaging the correct muscles, reduces strain on your joints, and prevents injuries. Here are some practical tips and guidance on correcting posture, particularly in the context of chair yoga.

First, choose the appropriate chair. To reduce the chance of it toppling over, your chair should be strong and level, preferably without wheels. Your knees should be bent to a 90-degree angle and your feet should be flat on the floor at the seat height. This alignment equally distributes your weight and aids in maintaining a neutral spine.

Sitting correctly on the chair is the foundation of good posture. Start by sitting towards the edge of the chair with your feet hip-width apart and flat on the ground. Ensure your weight is distributed evenly across both hips. Avoid slouching or leaning to one side, as this can cause imbalances and strain your muscles.

Engage your core muscles to support your spine. Think about gently drawing your navel in towards your spine. This engagement helps stabilize your lower back and prevents excessive arching or rounding of the spine. Your back should be straight but not rigid. Imagine a string pulling you up from the crown of your head, lengthening your spine, and encouraging a natural curve in your lower back.

Your shoulders play a significant role in maintaining good posture. Roll your shoulders up towards your ears and then back and down. This movement helps open up your chest and aligns your shoulders over your hips. Keep your shoulders relaxed and avoid tensing them, which can lead to neck and upper back discomfort.

Pay attention to your head and neck position. Your head should be aligned with your spine, not jutting forward or tilted back. Imagine a straight line running from your ears down to your shoulders and hips. To find the correct position, gently tuck your chin slightly and lengthen the back of your neck. This alignment reduces strain on your neck and upper back.

When performing chair yoga poses, always start with this aligned posture. Whether you are doing a seated twist, a forward bend, or a side stretch, maintaining this neutral alignment is crucial. For instance, in a seated forward bend, hinge at the hips while keeping your back straight rather than rounding your spine. This movement protects your lower back and ensures that the stretch targets the intended muscles.

Using props can be extremely beneficial in maintaining proper posture. A yoga block or cushion can provide additional support and help you maintain alignment in various poses. For example, placing a block between your knees can help keep your legs hip-width apart and engage your inner thighs, promoting stability. Similarly, a small cushion behind your lower back can support the natural curve of your spine and prevent slouching.

Breathing correctly also enhances your posture. Deep, diaphragmatic breathing not only relaxes your muscles but also supports your spine. As you inhale, allow your abdomen to expand, and as you exhale, gently contract your abdominal muscles. This breathing technique encourages the engagement of your core and supports your lower back.

Regularly checking your posture throughout your practice is important. Every few minutes, take a moment to reassess your alignment from head to toe. Ensure your feet are flat, your weight is evenly distributed, your spine is long, your shoulders are relaxed, and your head is aligned with your spine. Making these adjustments as needed helps reinforce good posture habits and prevents the development of poor alignment over time.

Consistency is key in developing and maintaining good posture. Practicing proper alignment in chair yoga will carry over into your daily life, helping you maintain better posture when sitting, standing, and moving throughout the day.

Being mindful of your posture outside of yoga practice is equally important. For example, when sitting at a desk, driving, or watching TV, apply the same principles of alignment to prevent strain and promote overall spinal health.

Strengthening the muscles that support good posture is another essential aspect. Chair yoga poses that target the core, back, and shoulder muscles can help build the strength needed to maintain proper alignment. Exercises like seated cat-cow stretches, chair twists, and seated shoulder rolls are excellent for strengthening these areas and promoting flexibility.

Incorporating stretching into your routine can also help improve posture. Tight muscles, particularly in the hips, hamstrings, and chest, can pull your body out of alignment. Regularly stretching these muscles can alleviate tension and support better posture. For instance, a seated hamstring stretch helps lengthen the muscles in the back of your legs, reducing the likelihood of pulling your pelvis out of its natural position.

Another helpful tip is to visualize good posture. Imagine a string running from the top of your head down to your pelvis, pulling you upward and keeping you aligned. Visualizations like this can help you maintain awareness of your posture and make necessary adjustments throughout your practice and daily activities.

Finally, practice mindfulness to enhance your posture. Being present and aware of how your body feels in different positions allows you to make conscious adjustments and prevent poor alignment. Meditation and mindful breathing practices can increase your overall body awareness, making it easier to maintain good posture naturally.

By following these tips and consistently practicing good posture in chair yoga, you can maximize the benefits of your practice. Proper alignment not only enhances the effectiveness of the poses but also protects your body from injury and promotes overall well-being. With time and practice, maintaining good posture will become second nature, contributing to better health and improved quality of life.

Video Tutorials

Scan this QR code to access the video tutorials

CONCLUSION

Reflecting on Your Journey

Embarking on a journey of self-improvement, particularly one that involves your health and well-being, is a profound endeavor that reshapes not just your physical body but also your mental landscape and emotional resilience. As you reach the end of this path or perhaps merely a rest stop along a much longer route, it's essential to pause and reflect on the progress you've made and the transformations you've undergone.

From the first tentative steps, where even small tasks or changes felt daunting, to a point where you now find a rhythm and ease in routines that once challenged you, your journey is worth acknowledging. Reflection is not merely about patting yourself on the back. It's about understanding how far you've come, recognizing the barriers you've overcome, and setting a course for where you want to go next.

Begin by recalling your initial motivations. What drove you to start this journey? Was it a desire to improve your physical health, reduce stress, enhance your mental clarity, or perhaps all of these? Think about those early days, the initial discomfort, and the perseverance it took to continue. Reflecting on these moments can reignite your motivation and help you appreciate the depth of your dedication.

Consider the changes in your physical health. Perhaps there's been weight loss, or maybe you've gained muscle tone or enhanced flexibility. Possibly, it's the endurance you've built up or the ease with which you now perform activities that once left you breathless. Each of these physical milestones is a testament to your commitment and the effort you've invested in your well-being.

But beyond the physical, reflect on your mental and emotional growth. Yoga and meditation, often parts of health journeys, not only transform the body but also bring about a greater sense of mental clarity and emotional stability. Have you noticed a decrease in stress levels? Are you better able to manage anxiety or find yourself more centered in the face of challenges? These are significant gains, signaling improvements in your overall quality of life.

Think about the skills you've developed, such as discipline from sticking to a workout regimen or mindfulness from practicing meditation. These skills often translate into other areas of life, improving your relationships, your work efficiency, and your ability to cope with unexpected difficulties. Reflection allows you to see the holistic improvement in your life brought about by your commitment to health.

It's also beneficial to acknowledge the support systems that have been part of your journey. Whether it's friends who joined you in workouts, family who encouraged you, or instructors who guided you, recognizing their contribution helps solidify your network of support. Gratitude for their roles in your journey not only deepens your relationships but also reinforces your support system for future challenges.

As you reflect, it's crucial to set new goals. With each accomplishment, new horizons may appear that were not visible when you started. Maybe now you feel ready to tackle a half-marathon, or perhaps you want to deepen your yoga practice with more advanced poses or explore meditation retreats. Setting new goals keeps the momentum of your journey going, pushing you to continue growing and evolving.

In your reflection, be honest about the setbacks as well. Every journey has its ups and downs; acknowledging the hurdles you encountered and how you overcame them (or are still working to overcome them) is integral to your growth narrative. These are not failures but part of the learning process, providing valuable lessons that strengthen your resilience.

Finally, take a moment to truly feel proud of what you've accomplished. Self-recognition is vital. It's not about ego but about acknowledging your own strength and perseverance. This acknowledgment is what builds self-esteem and confidence, propelling you forward.

Reflecting on your journey is a dynamic tool that not only gives depth to your past efforts but also shapes your future path. It turns abstract experiences into concrete achievements and lessons, framing your continuous journey not just in terms of health and fitness but as a lifelong quest for growth and fulfillment. As you move forward, carry these reflections as badges of honor and stepping stones to further achievements, knowing that every step you take is part of a larger tapestry of your life's journey.

Continuing Your Chair Yoga Practice

Engaging in a chair yoga practice is a commitment to improving your physical and mental well-being, and the benefits extend far beyond the time you spend on the mat. As you close this chapter of your yoga journey with the guidance of this book, it's essential to look forward to how you can weave the practices and principles of chair yoga into your everyday life. Continuing your chair yoga practice long-term can be one of the most rewarding decisions, providing a constant source of support and well-being.

The key to continuing your chair yoga practice is integration. This means finding ways to incorporate the movements and mindfulness you've learned into your daily routines. For example, consider starting your day with a few minutes of seated stretches. This can be done even before you leave your bed in the morning. Simple stretches such as reaching your arms above your head, twisting your torso from side to side, or doing some neck rolls can awaken your body gently and set a positive tone for the day.

Another effective way to integrate chair yoga into your daily life is by taking short yoga breaks throughout your workday. If you spend long hours at a desk, incorporating five minutes of chair yoga for every hour of sitting can significantly reduce stiffness and boost your energy levels. Simple poses like seated cat-cow stretches, torso twists, or forward bends can be done right at your desk. These movements not only help keep your body from feeling stagnant but also aid in maintaining focus and productivity.

You might also consider chair yoga as a tool for stress management. Whenever you feel overwhelmed or need a mental break, turn to your breathing exercises and gentle stretches. Deep, mindful breathing can be a powerful tool for calming the mind and reducing anxiety. You can practice this anywhere—at your desk, in your car, or even while waiting in line. The more you practice, the more natural it will become to use these techniques to manage stress in real time.

To keep your practice fresh and continually evolving, regularly seek out new chair yoga routines or variations. The internet is a rich resource, offering countless videos, tutorials, and articles that can introduce new poses and sequences. Engaging with online communities or local groups practicing chair yoga can also provide motivation and new ideas.

Setting personal goals related to your chair yoga practice can also keep you motivated. Perhaps you aim to master a particularly challenging pose or to practice for a continuous string of days. Maybe your goal is more about how you feel—such as achieving better sleep or managing a health condition like back pain. By setting and working toward these goals, your practice remains dynamic and personally relevant.

Another way to maintain your enthusiasm for chair yoga is by tracking your progress. Keep a journal of your practice, noting not only what you do each day but also how you feel physically and mentally afterward. Over time, reviewing this journal can provide visible proof of the benefits your practice is bringing, which can be incredibly motivating.

Consider teaching others what you have learned. Sharing your knowledge of chair yoga with friends, family, or colleagues can reinforce your own practice and provide additional motivation. Teaching is a powerful way to deepen your own understanding because it challenges you to think about and articulate what you know in new ways.

Finally, remember to celebrate your journey. Every so often, reflect on how far you've come since you began practicing chair yoga. Recognize the improvements in your flexibility, strength, and mental well-being. Celebrating these victories, no matter how small, can boost your motivation to continue.

Incorporating chair yoga into your daily life ensures that the practice is not just a temporary hobby but a lasting part of your routine. It becomes woven into the fabric of your daily activities, continuously contributing to your health and happiness. As you move forward, let chair yoga be your steady companion, adapting and growing with you as you navigate the complexities of life. Embrace it not just as an exercise but as a philosophy for living with awareness, grace, and vitality.

Dear Readers,

Thank you for completing this book. We hope that the chair yoga practices you've learned will continue to enhance your life. If you found the exercises and tips useful, please take a moment to leave a review on Amazon. Your feedback not only supports our work but also assists others in making informed decisions about their health and wellness choices.

How You Can Share Your Review

Through Amazon.com:

1. Go to the Amazon page where you found my book.

2. Navigate to the 'Customer Reviews' section.

3. Click on 'Write a customer review' to share your valuable insights.

Instant QR Code Access: Simply scan the QR code below with your smartphone to be directed to the Amazon review section.